Finding Effective
Acupuncture Points

Finding Effective Acupuncture Points

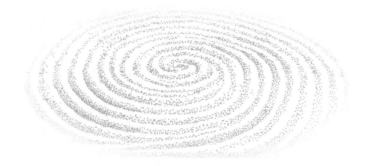

Shudō Denmei

TRANSLATED BY

Stephen Brown

EASTLAND PRESS • SEATTLE

Portions of this book were originally published in Japanese by
Ido-No-Nippon-Sha, Inc. as a series of journal articles between 1986 and 1990.

Published by Eastland Press, Incorporated
P.O. Box 99749, Seattle, WA 98199 USA

International Standard Book Number: 0-939616-40-8
Library of Congress Control Number: 2002113186

2 4 6 8 10 9 7 5 3 1

Book design by Gary Niemeier

TABLE OF CONTENTS

Points on the Leg and Foot 173

CHAPTER 3 **Effectively Treating Acupuncture Points**

FOREWORD

S HUDO DENMEI HAS DONE IT AGAIN. He has written a book that is easy to
read, easy to understand, packed full of information, and clinically invaluable.
This book reflects the same qualities that won Shudo the Manaka prize in Japan for
his first book *Keiraku Chiryo no Susume*, which is available in English from
Eastland Press under the title *Japanese Classical Acupuncture: Introduction to
Meridian Therapy*. His work has been, and continues to be, seminal. His clarity,
honesty, and openness are refreshing and invigorating.

This book, *Finding Effective Acupuncture Points*, might be described as a point-
location book, but it is much more than that. Shudo not only describes the location
of the points, but what they feel like when you look for them, how best to palpate
and find them, how to interpret the different reactions that you can palpate, how
best to treat them, and their most valuable clinical applications. If that were not
enough, he has also added a section describing treatment techniques, focusing in
particular on some rather sensitive needling methods.

The book primarily describes the use of acupuncture points in the relief of
symptoms, the *hyōji* or branch treatment. While not described much in this book,
elsewhere Shudo strongly emphasizes the importance of the *honji* or root treatment
in order to get better treatment results (see Shudo's *Japanese Classical Acupuncture:
Introduction to Meridian Therapy*). Thus, the recommended treatments in this
book are to be added to the root treatment for maximum effectiveness.

Yet summarizing the book in this manner understates the breadth of what Shudo
has done. By briefly comparing what is usually published about the acupuncture
points, the breadth and depth of what he has done here will become more readily
apparent.

Acupuncture point books typically describe the location of each point in anatomical terms. They describe the preferred methods of treatment, including the depth of needling and numbers of moxa cones to be applied. They also describe the particular qualities of each point, for example, that it is a luo-network vessel point, and then list the conditions for which the point is said to be most useful. Historically, there have been many such descriptions of the acupuncture points. The earliest ones usually left much room for interpretation, as they were often not very clear. Over time, other textbooks described the location, treatment methods, and uses of points differently. Not only did these differences reflect new attempts to explain or clarify the older descriptions, they also incorporated the experiences and ideas of later practitioners. Thus, over the centuries, the location, nature, uses, and recommended treatment methods of the acupuncture points evolved, and were often quite different.

In the modern period, however, especially in the West, much of the historical detail and variation among textbooks has been omitted as more definite and clear definitions and statements about the points have become the norm. Thus, students in acupuncture schools during the past century have learned precise anatomical locations for the points, specific methods for treating them, and very definitive statements about their nature and uses. Rarely are modern students shown the historical variety that preceded this certainty, and often students graduate from acupuncture schools in the belief that they *know* what the points are and how to use them. Rarely are they taught that these descriptions are modern summaries of previous ideas, or modern descriptions moulded into the model of practice that the students learned in school.

In other words, in the West students often come to believe that what they have learned is how the points have historically been described and thought about, as if there were an unaltered chain of information through a system of practice over the last two millennia. In short, very rigid and fixed ideas about the acupuncture points have developed in the modern period, especially in the West, where information is abbreviated through limited translation, or the absence of many translated texts.

By contrast, Japanese moxibustionists and meridian therapists in the first part of the twentieth century extensively read and studied the historical literature on acupuncture. Typical of the historical Asian way of processing information, these diverse descriptions were allowed to coexist side by side while practitioners explored them through clinical practice. Through these efforts, practitioners came to understand the acupuncture points as things that become active or alive when they need to be treated.

The *active point* is a concept that reputedly started with Takeshi Sawada, a famous moxibustionist, whose work Shudo himself learned and practiced before turning to meridian therapy. This concept has been picked up by the meridian therapy movement and is now common. One even finds that practitioners will refer to an anatomical point as being "dead," an anatomical landmark from which one starts searching for the "live" point. This reflects the need for some kind of palpable reaction when a point is to be treated. Of the more than forty Japanese acupuncturists that I have observed in Japan, none ever needled or treated with moxibustion a point that was not first palpated to determine its precise location, regardless of the school or style of acupuncture they practiced.

Palpation has become a sophisticated and refined art in the fields of acupuncture and moxibustion in Japan; it is emphasized much more there than in other countries. It is also quite common to find experienced practitioners practicing point location when they get together with other members of their particular association. In some, such as the Toyohari Meridian Therapy Association, point location is a study theme that is visited in virtually every monthly study-practice session.

For many who palpate to find the points that need to be treated, the location of points has evolved more into the idea of *point fields,* regions around a specific anatomical site within which one will generally find the reactive point if that point needs to be treated. Thus, point location has become a more flexible concept, not the fixed anatomical certainty that is taught in many modern acupuncture books. This not only reflects the work of practitioners who describe point locations based on their actual experience, it also allows the *variability* of historical ideas about point locations to be integrated flexibly into clinical practice, where it can be explored and tested.

This approach is preeminently practical and based on experience. Here the theoretical explanations for what is found and why those findings occur tend to be rather minimal, reflecting the minimum explanation needed for a clinician to use the approach within a treatment system. Hence, this approach fits well with the basic system of *keiraku chiryo*, or meridian therapy, that Shudo Denmei practices.

Shudo Denmei is obviously a master of this approach. In this book he describes many points, giving several typical locations at which the palpable reactions might be found, and citing various historical and modern texts to illustrate where these ideas probably came from. He describes his experiences of finding these variant point locations, the quality of the variant reactions, what he has found to be the best techniques for treating these reactions, and the medical conditions typically associated with them.

Like few others before it, this book confronts the uncertainty of clinical practice, giving the practitioner permission to examine the patient rather than dogmatically following some theory. It presents a wealth of experiences that move the reader away from uncertainty toward the more solid ground of observable and repeatable clinical experience. Shudo is usually very clear in recounting the commonly found locations of the palpably reactive points. He is also clear when those experiences rest on only one or two cases, as opposed to extensive or repeated experiences. His prioritization of the points in terms of how frequently he uses them is also invaluable. The book presents clear guidelines about probable selection of points by giving some order to the process of palpating to select those points that need to be treated.

While reading the manuscript in preparation for writing this foreword, I must admit that I have been applying in the clinic some of what Shudo Denmei has written. In most cases where I have tried something new based on what I just read, I found it clinically useful. This increases my confidence that those using this book will find it to be an invaluable and essential guide when treating patients. It should become a primary tool for anyone who palpates the body prior to administering acupuncture or moxibustion. In addition, it will help acupuncturists expand the effectiveness of their treatments, even if they have not yet been trained in the palpation-focused approaches that are characteristic of Japanese acupuncture.

In short, I heartily recommend this book to all practicing acupuncturists. If you are not yet familiar with this empirical, but highly-informed model of treating patients, and are accustomed to following a more theoretically driven model of practice, you will surprise yourself when you start using some of what is described here. For those already conversant with Japanese acupuncture and moxibustion treatment approaches *(ganbatte)*, we owe Shudo Denmei an increasing debt of gratitude for this excellent work. To Mr. Shudo: thank you for the honor of being asked to write a foreword to your excellent book.

Stephen Birch

PREFACE

SATISFACTORY RESULTS CAN BE obtained from an acupuncture treatment only when the four steps of diagnosis, point selection, point location, and needle insertion come together properly. Each of these steps is important, but palpating the point and inserting the needle are especially important and require many years of practice. Like any craft, even though it does take time, by practicing diligently every day, one eventually becomes proficient. I believe the time it takes to acquire these skills can be shortened if there is a suitable text that explains how to master certain techniques. This book is an attempt to do just that.

I have always been rather inept myself, and have often felt frustrated and dissatisfied. For a period of time, I even gave up on ever becoming skillful at point location and needling. Be that as it may, since I had no other occupation but acupuncture, I gradually began to acquire some skill as I applied myself in my practice. Acupuncture started to become fun once I learned to accurately locate active points and gained the ability to feel the arrival of qi. I have found that there is no limit to how much you can improve your technique. No matter how old you get, as long as you are alive and practicing, there is unlimited potential for improvement. Of course, this takes some effort. The point is to be persistent and to keep practicing.

Japanese Classical Acupuncture: Introduction to Meridian Therapy, the English edition of which was published over a decade ago, has been well received and is widely read. I believe this is because it presents meridian therapy in a simple and understandable way, and because Stephen Brown did an excellent job translating it. I am delighted that this book is being published under the same conditions, and I hope that it will be read for a long time to come. It is my sincere wish that the reader learn to locate points that are effective, thereby providing treatments that are satisfactory to both the patient and practitioner alike.

Finally, I would like to express my heartfelt thanks to Stephen Birch for his foreword, to Dan Bensky, medical editor at Eastland Press, for his enthusiasm in publishing my work, and to Stephen Brown for again serving as my translator.

Shudo Denmei

CHAPTER ONE

Acupuncture Points and Palpation

Introduction

T HE ACUPUNCTURE POINTS which I present in this text are only those which I use in my clinic on a regular basis. This makes the book quite different from the typical acupuncture point textbook, because it is based on a different standard. When I use acupuncture points that I learned about from my teacher, other acupuncturists, and textbooks, I sometimes find that their effects are not as stated. This could be because the point is not an active or 'living' point which manifests a reaction at that time, or it could be because my point location is off. In any case, when I don't get results, I stop using the point. Also, even though a book may list certain indications for a point, sometimes the point works unexpectedly for a condition I never knew it could help. I am surprised and elated when this happens.

Repeating this process of trial and error over the years, a group of points have become embedded in my mind and body. While it may be based on a biased and limited perspective, these points nonetheless have clinical significance in that they have been filtered through one acupuncturist's practice. Ever since I started writing *Japanese Classical Acupuncture: Introduction to Meridian Therapy*, it has been my policy to make sure that everything I write about has passed through the filter of my own experience. Therefore, in this text, the selection of points, judgments

1

about their relative value, location, insertion, and indications are all presented from this perspective.

It can fairly be said that this is a book about "Shudo's points," for it does not represent the general consensus about acupuncture points. Many practitioners and scholars have written texts on what is already well-established information about the acupuncture points, and I recommend that the reader consult such books if he or she is interested in the standard knowledge.

Before discussing individual acupuncture points, I would like to share some perspectives about acupuncture points in general, and explain the palpation technique I use to detect active or 'live' points *(ikita tsubo)*.

How Were Acupuncture Points Discovered?

When our shoulders get tight, our hands naturally go to our shoulders. We press, pinch, and pound on them, and may even apply some ointment. This is the beginning of "hands-on" healing, known as *te-ate* in Japan. It is even said that acupuncture points were discovered in this way. Why, then, is it that the meridians and acupuncture points were specifically discovered in China, and that for a time acupuncture was only practiced there?

I have thought of one possible scenario. The oldest document containing the word needle is the pre-Han classic *Spring and Autumn Annals: Zuo Commentary (Zuo shi chun qiu)* in which the characters *shitsu/zhí* (to hold in the hand) and *shin/zhēn* (needle) are used together. In this text, the word *shishin/zhí zhén* refers to a seamstress. The needles of acupuncture were no doubt derived from those used for sewing, and were adapted for therapeutic purposes. One thing that existed in ancient China, and nowhere else, was silk. Unlike the sari worn by Indian women, silk fabric was not loosely wrapped around the body. Silk fabric was of little use in the cold climate of China unless it was cut and sewed to fit the body. This is why the work of seamstresses was so important. Even today, when a person sews or knits for a long time, the muscles in the neck and shoulders become tense and begin to feel stiff. As the stiffness increases, many other symptoms such as heaviness in the head, headache, nausea, vomiting, fatigue, and insomnia begin to appear.

A seamstress experiencing these discomforts may have, without thinking about it, pressed her neck and shoulders in the vicinity of GB-20 and GB-21 with the needle still in her hand. It didn't really hurt to push the needle against the skin; in fact, she could hardly feel it. It even felt good to press a little bit harder. Increasing the pressure a bit more, she may have felt the sensation penetrate to the core of the shoulder tension, and also extend up her neck to the temples, and even to the center of her head. It may have been felt down her arms to her fingers, and even to the abdomen, causing her stomach to growl. Her headache then disappeared, and her head became clear. Suddenly, she came to herself, and, resuming her needle-work, noticed blood on the tip of her needle. She quickly wiped the blood off her shoulders, and for good measure, pressed down on the point to squeeze out any extra blood near the surface.

This may be taking things a little too far, but the location of acupuncture points and the effect of needling may have been learned in just this manner. Even more than the fact that certain points brought relief from symptoms, people may have noticed that there was an effect on places far removed from the point. Over time, and after many such points were discovered, they became organized and systematized. The meridians were probably formulated in this way. In any case, both the meridians and acupuncture points resulted from the keen insight, sensitivity, and clinical observation of the ancient Chinese.

It is said that the meridians were found after the acupuncture points were discovered. This seems only natural, since everything appears to progress from the simple to the complex. And yet the earliest texts on the subject list the names of meridians more often than individual acupuncture points. For example, the following passage appears on the silk manuscripts found at Ma Wang Dui in the 1970s: "When disturbed, disease occurs and there are palpitations, cardiac pain, and pain in the supraclavicular fossa . . . these can be treated on the greater yin meridian of the arm." (Shudo, 1990) This means that, for such-and-such symptoms, a certain meridian was treated. Once the appropriate meridian was determined, it was unnecessary to be too specific about which points to treat. It seems like a much simpler and smarter approach to place the emphasis on the meridians, and perhaps a particular meridian was chosen based on the reaction of a point or a set of points. Yet another way of looking at this is that in the early days, the location and indications of individual points were unclear. Whatever the case may be, the acupuncture points and meridians developed together, each supporting the other.

What are Acupuncture Points?

What are these acupuncture points which we use every day in our practices, as a matter of course? I would like to review what our predecessors said about them, then add my own comments, and organize the definitions.

"There are 365 qi holes which correspond to the [days of the] year." (*Basic Questions*, Chapter 54)

"The sites of treatment in acupuncture are called acupuncture points. There are countless acupuncture points on the body. But 'countless' leaves us nowhere, so 365 points were designated, applying the principle of correspondence between Heaven and Man.... In periods when the lunar calendar was used and 354 days were designated to a year, the number of standard points was likewise reduced to 354. The points given in *Elaboration of the Fourteen Meridians* are based on this [system]." (Araki, 1957)

Human beings are a microcosm that resonate with the macrocosm of the universe. The twelve meridians correspond to the twelve months of the year, and the 365 points correspond to the 365 days in the year. Yet the number of acupuncture points is not fixed. Among the standard points, some have fallen out of use, and new ones with clinical value (miscellaneous points and new points) have come into use. I think this transition from old to new will continue, and only those acupuncture points which are truly useful will remain in use.

. . . .

"All holes [acupuncture points] in the human body are places where qi resides." (Zhang, 1624)

"The meridians are channels for qi flow and the acupuncture points are gates along the channels." (Okabe, 1974)

Blood flows through the vessels, and qi circulates around and through them. In addition, blood accompanies the flow of qi. When qi stagnates, blood ceases to flow. The acupuncture points are places where the qi inside the body interfaces with the external environment. This is why the terms 'gate' or 'doorway' fit perfectly. It stands to reason that supplementing normal qi or draining pathogenic qi is done most effectively at the gates. Furthermore, when there is an overall deficiency of qi, these points are the most suitable places for absorbing yang qi.

. . . .

"The sun [travels] west and yang qi declines, and thus the gates of qi close." (*Basic Questions*, Chapter 3)

"These [acupuncture points] were considered to be places where the 'qi of Heaven' or 'yang qi' such as the atmosphere, heat, and the sun's rays were absorbed." (Yamashita, 1972)

"Qi transforms into qualities." (*Basic Questions*, Chapter 5)

4

"When one detects [the associated points of the five yin Organs] and wishes to test this, a response is obtained by pressing that place; it is inside and pain is relieved. This then is the point." (*Vital Axis*, Chapter 51)

"Acupuncture points are something which manifest only after there is repeated physical strain or fatigue and one is ill. They are not something that can be found on anyone at any time. If there is no illness, the meridians and points do not manifest." (Okabe, 1983)

Acupuncture points are hard to locate on healthy individuals. However, when qi stagnates or pathogenic qi invades from the outside, the point becomes depressed or protrudes. Qi, which is invisible, is thus transformed into a 'quality' that can be palpated and distinguished. This is what is known as an active point, which serves as both a point for diagnosis as well as treatment.

. . . .

"When there is disease in the five yin organs, there is a response, and it appears at the twelve source [points]." (*Vital Axis*, Chapter 1)

"It has been proven that there is a close relationship between tenderness at acupuncture points on the body surface and pathology of internal organs." (Gai, 1984)

Obviously, acupuncture points are related to the meridians, but we can also take the relationship between the five yin organs and the source points, mentioned in the first chapter of *Vital Axis*, one step further. According to Gai Guo-Cai in *Acupuncture Point Diagnosis*, certain points are related to specific internal organs, and can be linked clinically with specific diseases. Many of these points are not essential points, with five-phase or other associations. These are the so-called 'special effect points' or *tsubo*, a Japanese term meaning 'active point'.

From the foregoing discussion we can make the following conclusions:

1. Acupuncture points do exist.

2. Acupuncture points are gates along the course of meridians.

3. The qi in the meridians enters and exits through the acupuncture points.

4. Pathogenic qi can collect at acupuncture points.

5. The yang qi of heaven enters through the acupuncture points.

6. Changes on the inside of the body appear through these gates.

7. Pathology on the inside of the body can be detected through these gates; that is, they can be used for diagnosis. Applying treatment at these gates can correct internal problems; that is, they can be used for treatment.

8. There are some special connections between certain points and the internal organs.

In his groundbreaking book *Discourse on Meridian Therapy*, Honma Shohaku classified acupuncture points based on their application as follows: essential points that appear on all meridians, essential points that do not appear on all meridians, and other points. (Honma, 1949)

The essential points that appear on all meridians are the following:

1. Five-phase points (well, spring, stream, river, and sea)

2. Five essential points (source, connecting, cleft, front alarm, and back associated)

There are other important points that have systemic effects but do not appear on all the meridians, such as the eight confluence points and the lower uniting points.

As explained in my *Japanese Classical Acupuncture: Introduction to Meridian Therapy*, the effect of the five-phase points is quite amazing when they are used for the appropriate pattern *(shō)*. In fact, they work so well that the practitioner might fancy himself a master! Yet this is simply a result of unlocking the power behind the five-phase points.

As far as the other points are concerned, there are not as many rules about when and how to use them, but surprising results can be obtained when they are skillfully utilized. Most acupuncturists have a few such points in their repertoire, and the more such points that a practitioner has, the better he or she is at treatment. I want to discuss all these special points in the context of my own experience, but first I would like to talk about palpation technique, which is essential for locating the active or effective points.

How to Find Active Acupuncture Points

It is commonly believed in Japan that the key to success in acupuncture is finding and treating 'active points' *(ikita tsubo)*. There are many ways to translate this term in English, such as 'living' or 'reactive', but perhaps the most appropriate word is 'active'. This is because the opposite of active points are those which are dormant or inactive.

Active Points

Active acupuncture points manifest when there is some abnormality, but is there a rule for predicting when they will show up? It seems that there is a rule if one says there is, and there isn't if one says there isn't. We can say that the active points are often not the essential points. Beyond that, as you become more adept at point location, you will begin to detect some pattern in their occurrence, and thus will learn to locate them very quickly.

In reality, there are no rules regarding how or when they appear. Some points appear right on the surface, as if to say "Come on and needle me here!" Others are hiding next to a tendon or bone, while still other points seem to be holding their breath deep inside the body.

This is why detecting the points that will work best when used right now on the patient you are treating—the active acupuncture points—takes effort and ingenuity. We therefore need to use our patients as our textbook to continually study how to locate the most effective points. Remember that it was the acupuncture points themselves that came first, as points of reaction on ill bodies; textbooks about acupuncture points came later, as a description of this phenomenon. This is important. There are no hard and fast rules for finding acupuncture points. It is best to choose the method that works for you.

Points on the Surface

- *Points with abnormal temperature.* These are points that feel cooler or warmer than the surrounding area.

- *Depressed points.* These often appear in deficient patients. Some points are actually depressed, while for others it is the local qi that feels insufficient.

- *Points with abnormal moisture.* These points feel damper or drier (rougher) than the surrounding area.

- *Points with congestion (blood stasis).* These appear mostly on the abdomen. There is a peculiar sensation of softness or distention, as if pressing on an inflatable pillow.

Palpating points on the surface

Either the right or the left hand may be used. The following techniques for palpating the surface are difficult in the sense that they require special fingertip sensitivity.

- Stroke with the belly of the middle finger. The stroking can be up and down (vertical), back and forth (horizontal), or circular.
- Stroke with the belly of the index finger.
- Stroke with the belly of the thumb.
- Stroke with the middle finger together with others (two to four fingers).

Points Between the Surface and the Subcutaneous Tissues

The same techniques as described above are applied, but a little more pressure or a kneading action is used. I use the belly of my middle finger most often. I also use pinching, briefly reviewed below, to examine the skin and subcutaneous tissue.[1] Differences can be detected in the texture of the skin and subcutaneous adipose tissue by pinching the skin. Look for the following:

- Areas of skin that are thicker than others.
- Small lumps and nodules that can be felt by moving the thumb back and forth against the forefinger as the skin is pinched up.
- Points or areas that have a stinging sensation (hypersensitivity) when pinched.

Pinching techniques

- A *small pinch* is between the tips of the thumb and index finger.
- A *big pinch* is between the belly of the thumb and index finger. After pinching the skin, small circular movements can be made with the thumb to feel for differences. In this case, the index finger is not moved.
- To check a larger area, the index finger is bent into a "J" shape, and the middle phalanx and the thumb are used to pinch the skin. The thumb can be moved back and forth to feel for any differences (Fig. 1-1).

Pinching diagnosis was developed by Okabe Sodō as an extension of meridian palpation, but in my experience, findings of sensitivity to pinching seem to appear most often on the abdomen, especially along the Stomach meridian between ST-19 and ST-21. Findings of tenderness, induration, and sensitivity to pinching do not always appear together. Sometimes they appear at the same point, and at other times, independently. I believe it depends on the depth of the reaction.

Based on the location of the response to pinching on the abdomen, I surmise the existence of problems in the underlying visceral organs (Table 1-1). Of course, the correlation between location and the affected organ varies from patient to patient, but I find that they hold true in general.

Points in the Fascia and Muscle Tissue

You should palpate for indurations—that is, knots or areas of hardness—in the fascia and muscle tissue. Indurations come in many shapes including lines, circles, and other odd shapes. Therefore, it is sometimes difficult to distinguish the induration from the shape of the muscle itself.[2] The palpation techniques for indurated points are as follows:

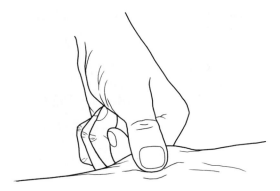

Fig. 1-1

Point	Organ
CV-12 and CV-14	Stomach and heart
Right LR-14	Liver
Right ST-19	Liver and gallbladder
Right ST-20	Gallbladder and liver
Right ST-21	Duodenum and gallbladder
Right ST-24	Duodenum
Left ST-19	Heart and stomach
Left ST-20	Stomach and pancreas
Left ST-21	Pancreas and stomach

Table 1-1

- Press with the tips of the thumb, index, and middle fingers, keeping the fingers straight.
- Bend the finger slightly, and press with the belly of the thumb, index, or middle fingers (Figure 1-2).
- Bend the distal joint and press the thumb vertically onto the skin. (Fig. 1-3), using the anterior surface of the thumb joint (Fig. 1-4).

In addition, there are several ways to move the finger(s):

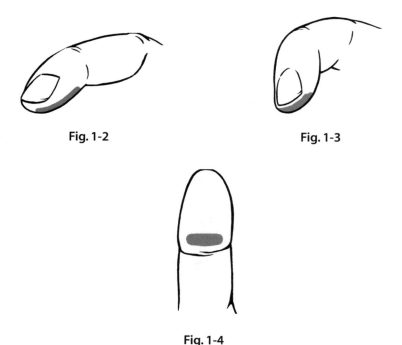

Fig. 1-2   Fig. 1-3

Fig. 1-4

- Apply vertical pressure to determine the borders of the induration.
- Apply a circular motion with the fingertip(s).
- Press and move up and down and sideways with a kneading motion.
- Hook and dig in with the fingertip(s), usually the thumb.

Points in Deeper Tissues

Sometimes points in the abdomen, lower back, or hips can be quite deep. Care must be taken when using more pressure because excessive pressure can cause discomfort and aggravate the pain. Firmly pressing on the abdomen, one can sometimes find hard areas in various places. Lighter palpation is adequate for traditional abdominal diagnosis, but I go one step further. I also palpate from a Western biomedical perspective, my aim being to detect pathological changes in the visceral organs.[3] To do this, I press my fingers deep into the abdomen to detect inflammation or hypertrophy of organs like the liver and gallbladder. To palpate these organs, I press four fingers firmly in under the right rib cage. In this way, I can detect abnormalities in the underlying tissues. Sometimes the reaction is quite strong and it does not take much pressure to get a response of tenderness or to feel the resistance.

I also like to use percussion when checking for reactions in the following underlying tissues:

- *Abdomen.* Use the standard Western biomedical technique for palpating internal organs, that is, press deeply into the abdomen with two to four fingers. Alternatively, one hand can be placed over the area, and this can be percussed lightly with the other hand.
- *Areas other than the abdomen.* Press firmly with the tip of the middle finger or thumb. When the location of a reaction or tender point is unclear even with the use of strong pressure, try percussion. I form a loose fist and strike with the knuckle of the little finger. Watch for the patient's reaction or facial expression.

Appropriate Amount of Pressure

Whenever palpating for a point, the less force that is used, the better. This applies regardless of the depth at which we palpate a point, but it is especially true for tender or indurated points. When we use excessive pressure, every place we press might seem like a tender point.

The term *monjun (mén xún)* appears in *Basic Questions* and *Vital Axis* now and then. *Mon* means to stroke lightly and *jun* has a similar meaning. In practice, to find the location of acupuncture points, we do not apply strong pressure, but tend to stroke the skin surface lightly to feel for something catching on (or sticking to) our fingertips. Also in *Vital Axis* is the passage "When depressed, apply moxibustion." Most likely the *monjun* technique was used to detect such depressions. That is to say, in *Basic Questions* and *Vital Axis*, strong pressure is used to determine the point of treatment only for pathology of the meridian sinews. Maruyama observes:

> Furthermore, the concept of tonification and dispersion are excluded in cases of sinew or muscle pathology. It therefore seems that tender (or tight) points are used for the treatment of meridian sinews and that the basic characteristics of other acupuncture points do not correspond to this. It seems only natural, therefore, that there should be a difference of opinion between the Sawada style, which aims at the treatment of tender points, and meridian therapy, which treats the other acupuncture points. (Maruyama, 1977)

My teacher practiced the Sawada style, which is noted for tender point treatment, but he did not use such strong pressure to palpate points. On one occasion,

11

when he visited Tokyo, he went to see Dr. Shiroda Bunshi, the leader of the Sawada style. Dr. Shiroda squeezed LI-4 on my teacher's hand with great force and said, "You are tired. HT-7 will take care of it." Even though my teacher had great admiration for Dr. Shiroda, he seemed perplexed and commented, "I really do not know why he had to press that hard."

Different Approaches to Palpation

Palpation techniques for the abdomen, meridians, and points are subtly different. To palpate the meridians, I like to gently stroke in the direction of the meridian flow using my middle finger, middle and index fingers, or middle, index, and ring fingers. I do this palpation primarily around the source points to determine or confirm the basic pattern. I do not press points to look for tenderness in this case.

This gentle stroking of the meridian is gradually transformed into gentle stroking for the purpose of point location. I use the same basic approach, but begin to focus on specific points, for example, LR-8 or LR-3 in cases of Liver deficiency. I generally use my middle finger to gently stroke the meridian and locate the most depressed point.

I use a different technique, however, to locate points on yang meridians. Points on the Gallbladder and Bladder meridians that I use often tend to be excessive. Therefore, I look for points that are tight or hard (indurations). I stroke along the yang meridians and gently press specific points. For example, on the Gallbladder meridian, I generally check GB-34, GB-38, and GB-41. Usually I find the most reactive (indurated) point on the meridian, and needle that point. All this is to say that I rarely go through the step of discriminating and treating deficiency and excess in the yang meridians.

Palpation as part of abdominal diagnosis is slightly different. When I am trying to confirm the underlying deficiency, as I have detailed in *Japanese Classical Acupuncture: Introduction to Meridian Therapy*, I use the palm of my right hand to lightly stroke the abdomen and chest, looking for depressed or tense areas. My touch is very soft. In my early years, I used to apply more pressure whenever I palpated, but over time I realized that one must palpate the meridians very gently in order to detect changes in the qi. This also applies to abdominal diagnosis, where gentle stroking is best for detecting changes in the qi. The palpation technique on the abdomen that I use today for determining the pattern is very gentle and quick—a few quick brushes over the abdomen.

Is this all that one needs to do when palpating the abdomen? I do not think so. After we have palpated for changes in the qi, we should palpate for changes in the blood (the structure). In meridian therapy, changes in the blood refer to indurations and areas of tension or fullness. Firmly pressing on the abdomen, one can find hard areas here and there. This is adequate for traditional abdominal diagnosis, but I go one step further, as indicated above; that is, I also palpate from a so-called modern medical perspective with the aim of detecting pathological changes in the viscera. In this way, I can provide a more complete diagnosis.

ENDNOTES

1. See *Japanese Classical Acupuncture: Introduction to Meridian Therapy,* p. 102, for a fuller discussion of this technique.

2. Ibid., 168-70.

3. Information on biomedical approaches to the abdominal exam can be found in such books as Barbara Bates, *A Guide to Physical Examination and History Taking.* Philadelphia: J.B. Lippincott Company, 1991.

CHAPTER TWO

The Acupuncture Points I Use

How to Use This Point Location Guide

IN THE FOLLOWING DISCUSSION, I will mention only those points I actually use in my practice. To indicate the frequency of use, one to three stars will be placed after the WHO designation or miscellaneous name of each point. Three stars (★★★) represents a point that I use quite often, one star (★) represents a point that I use once in a while, and two stars (★★) indicates a usage somewhere between one and three. This is not to say that any of these points is more effective in general than others. Each point is most effective when it is a clearly manifesting active point. Three stars simply indicates that a reaction tends to appear often and is easy to detect; when this is the case, the point works well. Therefore, one can say about the points that ★★★ > ★★ > ★ in terms of overall usefulness in my clinic.

The sequence of the points in this text follows that found in *Clarification of Acupuncture Points* (Hara, 1807). However, new points, miscellaneous points, and my own special points are included wherever it seems appropriate. Each entry begins with textual references concerning the location of the point. For this purpose, I used *Clarification of Acupuncture Points* most often. Thus, *Systematic Classic of Acupuncture and Moxibustion* (Huang-fu, 259), on which the above text is based, is the primary classical reference for my point location. A passage quoted from this text is preceded by the notation *(Systematic)*. Four other oft-quoted textbooks are listed under the "Primary References" section at the end of the Bibliography, with their key words underlined. I draw from many other sources as well, but for these occasional references, the author and date of publication, rather than the title, are listed in front of the quotation. For the oldest classics, like the *Yellow Emperor's Inner Classic,* I list only the English name for the cited text. In quoting from some texts, I have changed the wording slightly for greater clarity, being careful not to alter the original meaning. Note that words in brackets are added in the English translation to improve readability.

I use the following format in discussing each point:

- (REFERENCES): Passages quoted from a variety of textbooks regarding the location of the point.

- LOCATION: The location I use in my practice, which is based on these references.

- PALPATION: The way I palpate and locate the point in my practice.

- INSERTION: Considerations for needling or treating the point are described here. (The meaning of such terms as 'shallow' and 'superficial' are explained in the "Needles and Techniques" section in Chapter 3.)

- INDICATION: The condition or conditions for which the point is used are listed in this section. In my experience, the less frequently a condition is listed in a textbook, the easier it is to remember. I do not list all of the possible symptoms that a point may be used for, because things become very simple once you determine the primary pattern. All of the indications found in textbooks become much easier to apply when we categorize and understand them in this manner.

- DISCUSSION: Interesting stories regarding my own knowledge and experience with the point.

POINTS ON
THE CRANIUM

GV-23 *(jō-sei / shàng xīng)* ★★

(SYSTEMATIC): "Above the forehead in the center, straight above the bridge of the nose. One unit above the hairline, in the depression, a place just large enough to fit a bean.

LOCATION: On the midline, one unit above the hairline (Fig. 2-1).

PALPATION: Stroke along the midline from the hairline toward the vertex with the tip of the middle finger. The finger will come to a stop in a depression; it is tender when pressed. Sometimes, there will instead be a protrusion. Circle with the fingertip to locate this point.

INDICATION: For nasal discharge, use 5 to 7 cones of direct moxibustion, and for acute conditions such as colds, 10 to 15 cones can be applied. Moxibustion can be applied at this point by the patient using a mirror, so GV-23 is a good point for home treatment. As for acupuncture, I sometimes use this point instead of GV-22.

DISCUSSION: When a person's hairline is distinct, this point is easy to locate. Sometimes, however, there is no hairline at all, and it is impossible to locate. What can be done in such cases? The following approaches are useful:
    "The distance from the point between the eyebrows to GV-14 is divided into 18 units. The anterior hairline is two-and-a-half units above the point between the eyebrows, and the posterior hairline is three-and-a-half units above GV-14." (Honma, 1955)
    "When hair has been lost and [the hairline] is not clear, designate the anterior hairline as being three units above [the point] between the eyebrows." (Manase, 1578)
    "As a convenient way of locating this point, place the heel of the palm over the

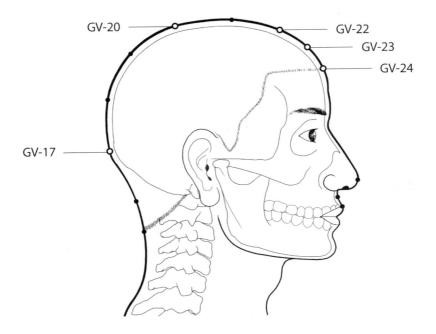

Fig. 2-1

point between the eyebrows and then press the scalp with the tip of the little finger. This will correspond exactly to the depression of GV-23. Pressing this point will cause a sensation to radiate to the nose. Applying moxibustion here produces a penetrating sensation which will reach the nose." (Irie, 1980) (Fig. 2-2)

The last of the methods described above, suggested by the early twentieth–century moxibustion master Fukaya Isaburo, is the simplest one. This location is actually closer to GV-22, but when a person is bald and the original hairline is not clear, there rarely seems to be a reaction at GV-23. When there is no reaction, it is not an active point.

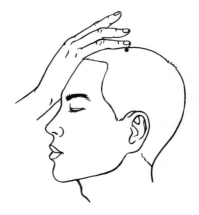

Fig. 2-2

GV-22 (*shin-e / xìn huì*)

(*SYSTEMATIC*): "One unit posterior to GV-23, between the bones, inside the depression. It is also known as *dīng mén* [crown gate]."

LOCATION: On the midline between GV-20 and the anterior hairline (Fig. 2-1).

PALPATION: Go from GV-20 to the center of the anterior hairline, pressing every third of an inch when there is thick hair. When the hair is thin or the person is bald, stroke down the center. You will find a point in a depression that, when pressed, is soft and sensitive. Locate this point with the tip of your middle finger. Move it back and forth or in a small circular motion. Do not be concerned about the standard location because this point moves quite a bit. While it often moves anteriorly or posteriorly, it does not move off the median line. Treatment at this point is not indicated when there is no depression and it feels hard, like a piece of wood. For infants under one year, a pulsation can be felt at this point. Pressing this point, not to mention needling, is forbidden in infants.

INSERTION: I use a 40mm, No. 1 or 0, stainless steel needle, pointing the tip of the needle toward the nose. The needle can be retained just after breaking the skin, or after a very shallow insertion (about one-fifth of a unit). Rotate the needle, and wait for the arrival of qi before retaining the needle. An intradermal needle can be retained here for twenty-four hours. When the patient has a strong headache, nausea, vomiting, or dizziness, however, I do not retain the needle. Instead, I do a simple insertion, rotating the needle and adding a slight, almost imaginary, pecking motion. Thick needles must not be used at this point. Excessive stimulation can cause hypotension and dizziness. Another way to stimulate the point is to use a plum blossom needle or to hold three Chinese needles between the thumb and index finger and lightly tap the points.

INDICATION: For dizziness it is best to retain the needle. For a chronic case of dizziness, three to five small cones of moxa can be applied. Other indications are headache, nausea, forgetfulness, insomnia, and the prevention and treatment of senility.

DISCUSSION: Not long after I opened my practice I was asked to make a house call for a 70-year-old woman who was a friend of my mother's. Since her youth, this patient experienced dizzy spells whenever she got tired. She was unable to get up that day, and when I got to her house I found her lying on her side with her eyes closed. I had given her treatments from time to time, and it seemed like she was improving, so I proceeded with the treatment. I do not know what got into to me, but I inserted a No. 10 needle into GV-22 and retained it. All of a sudden, she covered her face with her hands and shortly thereafter passed out. This patient had a history of strokes, so I cut the treatment short and told her family members to take her to a doctor. Fortunately, she recovered without incident, but I am really ashamed when I think back on this. I should have known that people with recurrent vertigo are hypersensitive, and only thin needles should be used in treating them. I thoughtlessly used a thick needle on this patient and aggravated her condition.

GV-20 (hyaku-e / bǎi huì)   ★

(SYSTEMATIC): "In the center of the crown, in the middle of the spiral of hair. A depression into which a finger fits."

(ELABORATION): "Straight above the top end of the ears."

(ACUPUNCTURE): "The midpoint between the external occipital protuberance [GV-17] and the center of the anterior hairline [GV-24]."

(GE, 340): "In the middle of the depression at the vertex."

LOCATION: At the intersection of the median line and the line connecting the top of the ears when they are folded forward (Fig. 2-1).

PALPATION: There is often a depression at the top of the head which, when pressed, is painful or tender. This point is indicated when it feels soft or spongy (a localized circulatory problem). When it feels hard, like pressing on a piece of wood, it is better to use a different point. This point is palpated by rocking the tip of the middle finger back and forth. Another way to locate GV-20 is to place the middle fingers in the openings of the ears, and then place both thumbs together on the crown. The reaction generally appears posterior to the standard location.

INSERTION: Retain the needle superficially at an angle, with the tip pointing forward.

INDICATION: GV-20 is effective for dizziness. I retain a needle at GV-20 for such cranial symptoms as headaches when I find the reaction is greater than what I find at GV-22. It therefore serves as an alternative to GV-22. Direct moxibustion at this point is effective for hemorrhoids.

DISCUSSION: Some texts recommend bloodletting for soft points on the crown. I once used a three-edged needle to bleed GV-20 on an elderly woman who had high blood pressure and edema. Some points on her head were so soggy that pressing left an indentation. I thought bloodletting would work, but contrary to my expectations, the patient became light-headed and asked me not to do it anymore. I have had several other experiences like this, which has led me to conclude that it is not good to intentionally bleed GV-20. It is best when it happens unexpectedly, that is, when you discover a drop or two of blood after removing a needle.

Some patients have remarked after treatment that retaining the needle in GV-20 felt uncomfortable. I once had a couple and their son come for treatment, and on separate occasions they told me that the stimulation of GV-20 felt uncomfortable. Retaining a needle caused a prickling sensation, and moxibustion left an uncomfortable hot sensation. When a person has high blood pressure, it is best not to do moxibustion on the head. Home moxibustion therapy should also be discouraged. For such patients we may burn very small cones on the back or on the limbs, but the cranial area should only be treated with acupuncture. I have read of a case where the use of moxibustion at GV-20 caused bleeding of the retinal vessels. The following passage appears in *Guide to the Secrets of Acupuncture*:

> If moxa is applied carelessly and excessively, qi will rise up [to the head] to cause nosebleeds, eye disease, or manic episodes. Seven cones may be applied only for those who are cold and deficient, where yang qi is deficient. Excessive [moxibustion] is to be avoided. (Okamoto, 1685)

According to an ancient Chinese legend, when the prince of the state of Guo was ill and became unconscious, Bian-Que inserted a needle at GV-20 and revived him. This is known in Japan as "a needle in the crown gate" *(chomon-no-isshin/dǐng mén zhī yī zhēn)*, and it means hitting the nail on the head. "Crown gate" is actually just another name for GV-22. I regard the midline on the crown, from just behind GV-20 to GV-23, to be a zone for treatment in which all points have the same effect as long as the point is active.

GV-16 (*fū-fu / fēng fǔ*)

(SYSTEMATIC): "On the crown, one unit above the [posterior] hairline, between the large tendons, in the middle of the big depression. When speaking, these tendons stand right out, and when speaking stops, they go back down. Moxibustion is forbidden."

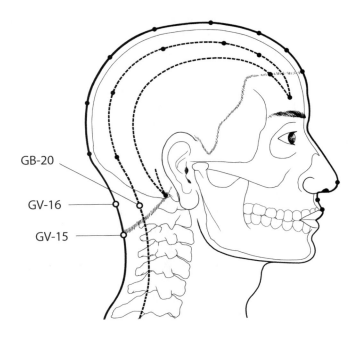

Fig. 2-3

LOCATION: Where the fingertip comes to a stop when the midline is stroked superiorly from the posterior hairline. Directly below the external occipital protuberance (Fig. 2-3).

PALPATION: Move the fingertip along the depression from side to side between the tendons to locate the deepest part of the depression.

INSERTION: Needle 0.2-0.3 unit diagonally and superiorly.

INDICATION: Epistaxis, nasal congestion, cases where needling BL-10 does not relieve neck tension.

GV-15 (*a-mon* / *yǎ mén*)

(*SYSTEMATIC*): "On the posterior hairline in the middle of the big depression. Internally, it connects to the root of the tongue. Insert 0.4 units. Do not apply moxa.

When moxa is applied at this [point], some will become mute."

LOCATION: Half a unit below GV-16 (Fig. 2-3).

PALPATION: There is a tender point between the vertebrae just below GV-16.

INSERTION: Insert vertically 0.3 to 0.5 unit, with the patient in a seated or prone position.

INDICATION: Aphasia, extreme headaches, facial pain.

DISCUSSION: Regarding this point, *Classification of the Classics* (Zhang, 1624) warns "Deep insertion is prohibited." Deep insertion at GV-15 supposedly causes loss of speech. Perhaps the ancients experienced many cases in which needling the occipital region caused aphasia. One must therefore be careful here, especially in cases of cerebrovascular accident. I have treated many patients who suffered recent strokes that caused paraplegia and speech impairment. The sooner that treatment is begun after the onset of paralysis, the better the chances for recovery.

Acupuncture treatment can even be started on the same day as the stroke. Treatment in the occipital area, however, is a different matter, for it often exacerbates the symptoms. The association between GV-15 and aphasia must have come from this concern. Limit the treatment to points on the arms and legs for the first few days. After that, points on the top of the head and auricular points can be added, but thin needles should be used. Also, be sure to use the auricular aphasia point. Try to get the patient to speak while the needles are retained in the aphasia point and points on the limbs. That way, their symptoms can be resolved more quickly. If a patient's progress is good, GV-15 can be used after the tenth day, but be sure to keep the insertion shallow.

BL-3 *(bi-shō / méi chōng)*

(SYSTEMATIC): "On the [anterior] hairline, half a unit to either side of GV-24."

LOCATION: Directly above BL-2, 0.5 unit above the hairline (Fig. 2-4).

PALPATION: Slide the tip of the middle finger superiorly, from the anterior hairline straight above BL-2. After finding a slight depression, circle the fingertip to find the tender point.

INDICATION: Five cones of direct moxibustion for excessive lacrimation and dacryocystitis (inflammation of the lacrimal glands).

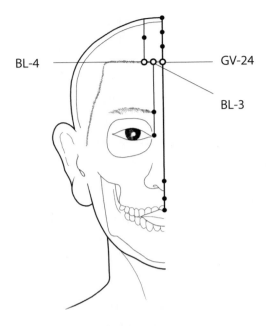

Fig. 2-4

BL-10 (*ten-chū / tiān zhù*)

(SYSTEMATIC): "On either side of the nape of the neck along the posterior hairline; in the depression on the lateral border of the great tendons."

(ILLUSTRATED): "Lateral to the tendon of the trapezius in the depression at the hairline."

LOCATION: In the tendon of the insertion of the trapezius muscles on the hairline (Fig. 2-5).

PALPATION: Often there is marked tenderness at the point where the trapezius muscle begins. This reaction can be found at the standard location for BL-10, but be sure to select the point with the strongest reaction.

INSERTION: Insert vertically 0.3 to 0.5 unit. Keep the insertion very shallow in patients with cerebrovascular problems. Merely retaining the needle after breaking the skin (2 to 3mm) is effective for such patients (see GV-15 above).

INDICATION: Stiff neck, headache, high blood pressure, and any symptom above the shoulders, goiter, sore throat, nasal congestion, whiplash, cervical syndrome, and 'cricks' in the neck. Bleeding just a few drops from this point is effective when there is strong tension in the occipital area and vascular 'spiders.' I do not, however, use BL-10 as often as points like GB-12, GB-20, and Upper BL-10.

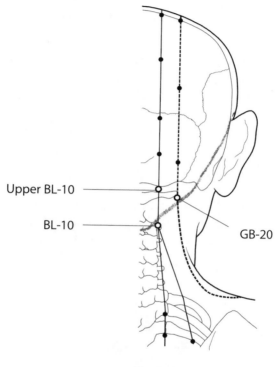

Fig. 2-5

Upper BL-10 [N-HN-44] (*kami-ten-chū* / *shàn tiān zhù*) ★★★

LOCATION: At the insertion of the trapezius on the occiput. BL-10 is on the trapezius at the hairline, and Upper BL-10 is one to 1.5 units superior to that point (Fig. 2-5).

PALPATION: When pressing the occiput where the tendon of the trapezius attaches, tenderness can be detected in three places: the center of the tendon (press superiorly), the medial side of the tendon (press laterally), and the lateral side of the tendon (press medially). The most tender point is usually on the lateral side of the tendon (Fig. 2-6).

INSERTION: I recommend shallow insertion (just breaking the skin) for patients who are new to acupuncture and those who are very sensitive, have high blood pressure, or cerebrovascular problems. Insert to a depth of 0.3 to 0.5 unit for other patients. Many people report a pleasurable sensation when you hit this point just right.

INDICATION: For any symptom in the upper half of the body. Use this point when the brain is overstimulated or excited. In this age of high stress, I use it on almost all my patients. It is also useful for neck and shoulder stiffness, headache, eye diseases, gynecological problems, perimenopausal syndrome, and urinary incontinence. I also apply direct moxibustion in cases of occipital neuralgia.

DISCUSSION: When patients complain of tension in the back of their neck and I have them show me where it is, most often they point to GB-20, followed by Upper BL-10; they point to BL-10 less often. When they are not sure, and I look for the point, in addition to the above points, I discover the focus of tension to be GB-12 or Yanagiya's GB-20 (see two points below). There is an indescribable sensation when the needle tip reaches the actual focal point, which causes a person to cry "That's it!"

Occiput

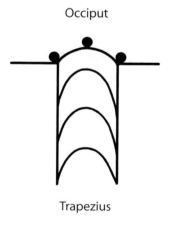

Trapezius

Fig. 2-6

GB-20 (*fū-chi / fēng chí*)   ★★★

(*BASIC QUESTIONS*): "On either side of GV-16."

LOCATION: In the depression midway between the trapezius and sternocleido-mastoid muscles (Fig. 2-5). An inverted triangle is formed by Upper BL-10, the tip of the mastoid process, and GB-20 (Fig. 2-7).

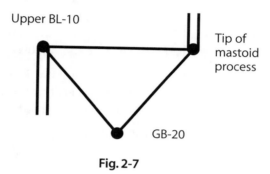

Fig. 2-7

PALPATION: To locate GB-20 on the left side, position yourself behind the patient, who is seated on the table. Place the thumb of your right hand lateral to BL-10 in the depression midway between the trapezius and sternocleidomastoid muscles. Place your index finger in the depression on the other side, with the other fingers below it. Probe for the point using your right thumb, using the four fingers on the opposite side for support. Hook the thumb and move it in small circles to locate tight bands and indurations. Press medially and superiorly. This point sometimes appears on the lateral side of the depression, that is, in the posterior border of the sternocleidomastoid muscle. When it does, it is best located by small front-to-back (cross-fiber) movements with the tip of the thumb.

To locate GB-20 on the right side, press with your left thumb and support the opposite side with the four fingers. When the patient is lying face down, I often stand at the head end of the table and use my middle finger to probe for the point. Sometimes I stand to the right of the patient's head and use my thumbs to locate the point. When the fingertip comes across the induration or tight point, the patient often feels a strong sensation reaching up to the temples or the top of the head.

27

INSERTION: Aim the needle anteriorly and slightly superiorly. When the tip of the needle reaches the hard point, it will produce a sensation that goes to the center of the head, the back of the eyes, or the temples. When the patient is new to acupuncture, this point should be needled in a face-down or side-lying position. If the patient is familiar with acupuncture, it can be needled in the seated position.

Special care must be taken in needling GB-20 because the vertebral artery, which connects with the basilar artery, lies under this point. Extra caution is needed when there is arteriosclerosis, which means in all elderly patients, and in cases of cerebrovascular disease. For patients who are new to acupuncture or who have cerebrovascular disease, just tap the needle in with the tube but do not insert it any deeper. For patients who are familiar with acupuncture, I insert the needle to a depth of 0.2 to 0.3 unit. Intradermal needles are also effective.

INDICATION: I often use GB-20 for any symptom above the shoulders. It is especially useful for symptoms in the cranium, eyes, and nose, as well as for stiffness in the neck and shoulders. This is a point with broad applications.

DISCUSSION: The literal translation of this point's name is 'wind pond' because it was thought to be an area where wind collected. It is interesting that there are several points whose names include the character for wind on the neck and shoulders. The ancients must have thought that external wind entered at this part of the body. They also thought that wind could then travel in three directions: above and below by way of the Bladder meridian; down the sides by way of the Gallbladder meridian; and downward from the face by way of the Stomach and Large Intestine meridians.

It is true that in the early stages of a cold, the upper back and neck feel chilled or uncomfortable. In this case, if contact needling or very shallow insertions are applied all over the area, it causes sweating, and the cold is quickly cured. Still, one should always be careful when needling in this area.

Shortly after I began my practice I made a house call to an elderly man with dizziness and pain in the occipital area. He was told when he went to a local hospital that is was probably just a cold. It crossed my mind that these might be pre-symptoms of a stroke, so I checked his blood pressure and reflexes. I found nothing out of the ordinary and so I gave him a regular treatment. When I went to see him again several days later, I was told he had fallen unconscious in the bathroom and was taken to the hospital. He had a stroke. I *could* say that I trusted the diagnosis at the hospital, or that I was still inexperienced. But no matter how you view it, the consequences of treating the occipital area can be very serious if one is not careful.

Some patients present with considerable tension or stiffness in the occipital area. It is not wise to treat points in the occipital area directly under the assumption that reducing the tension here will have a beneficial effect on cerebral circulation. There are many ways to alleviate such tension. The first and most effective way is to perform a root treatment, as done in meridian therapy. In this case, it is especially important to balance the yang meridians. Treating the Bladder, Gallbladder, and Large Intestine meridians has a marked effect. The second option is to use the back associated points, Governing vessel points, the eight *ryo/liáo* (sacral foramina) points (BL-31 to BL-34), and last but not least, the auricular points, which are very useful for this purpose. In my experience, needling the occiput points on the ear quickly reduces tension in the occipital area. According to the master of moxibustion, Fukaya Isaburo (1966), "It is the very worst approach to apply moxa to points simply because that is where the problem is."

This holds true for acupuncture as well. There are times when treatment is necessary at that very spot, but it is a problem when that is our only strategy. For the best results, one must know how to treat distally as well as locally.

Yanagiya's GB-20 (*yanagiya fū-chi*)   ★★★

This is a miscellaneous point introduced in *Guide to Secret One-Needle Technique* (Yanagiya, 1955) (Fig. 2-8). It is listed there as "No. 6, the point for all eye problems." This book discusses 'special effect points' that resolve symptoms with just one needle.

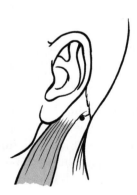

Fig. 2-8

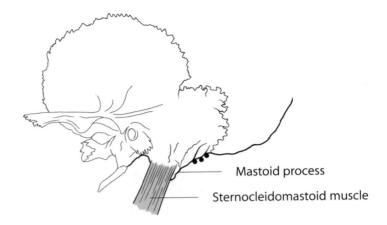

Mastoid process

Sternocleidomastoid muscle

Fig. 2-9

LOCATION: There is a small protuberance posterior and superior to the mastoid process. The protuberance is triangular and the tip points downward. It feels like cartilage or a so-called 'hard knob.' One point near this protuberance is most sensitive. Pressing it causes a strong sensation that extends to the temples (Fig. 2-9). This is in the area of the new Chinese acupuncture point from the 1960s known as N-HN-22(b) *(ān mián #2b).*[1]

PALPATION: Press the border of the occiput with the middle finger to locate the protuberance. Move medially from the back of the mastoid process, or laterally from the insertion of the trapezius (Upper BL-10). Locate this point on the tip of the 'peninsula' or in the depression on either side of it. Choose the most tender point, which often appears on the posterior border. It is easiest to locate with the patient lying on her side. Position yourself behind the patient and press superiorly with your middle finger as you rotate it slightly.

INSERTION: Position yourself behind the patient who is in the side-lying position. Face the patient's head and point the needle tip in a medial and superior direction, at a diagonal toward the opposite eyeball. According to Yanagiya (1955), "The right depth is reached between one-and-one-half and two units, when the needle sensation extends to the temples or the back of the eyes."

There will be no needle sensation if the needle enters without any resistance. Should this occur, remove the needle and reinsert until it meets resistance. I use a

40mm, No. 1 or 0, stainless steel needle and insert it only to the depth where it meets resistance.

INDICATION: As Yanagiya suggested, this point is good for eye problems. It is especially effective for lesions on the surface of the eye. Thus, it is fantastic for minor injuries or blows to the eye. It is also effective for ocular congestion and excessive tearing, and to improve the eyesight. Otherwise it is used for diplopia (double vision) caused by paralysis in the ocular motor nerve, and for headaches, especially lateral headaches, migraines, and occipital headaches. I also use it for *katakori*, that is, stiffness in the neck and shoulders.

DISCUSSION: It is common knowledge that GB-20 is effective for eye problems, but Yanagiya's GB-20 is even more effective. It could be regarded as a variation of GB-20 or GB-12, but given its effects, it deserves to be treated as an independent point. One of the early meridian therapists, Baba Hakkō, designated GB-20 as the premier point for improving vision. He taught that the needle should not be inserted into the induration, but should be retained as soon as it reached the surface of the induration. Eyesight should show improvement when it is checked while the needle is retained. Since learning this technique from Hakko, I have been applying it to Yanagiya's GB-20 and use it as my main point for improving vision. I once treated a man who failed his vision test twice when trying to renew his driver's license. He was very grateful when he was able to pass after just one treatment.

Injuries to the eyes were once common in farming communities of Japan. In the old days, people had to pick weeds by hand in the rice paddies, which required that they stoop over. Sometimes a farmer would get poked in the eye with the tip of a rice plant leaf. These leaves are very sharp, and their edges are rough and can cut like a razor blade. Thus, it can easily injure the eyeball and cause an infection. An eye infection is frightening because it not only impairs one's vision but can also lead to blindness. I was once visited by a patient with this condition, who was at a loss because visits to the ophthalmologist were not helping. Right after I needled Yanagiya's GB-20, the pain disappeared, and the next day the inflammation subsided. In this way, I have had dramatic results with this point. My teacher also used Yanagiya's GB-20 for cataracts, but the effect is not as fast as for problems on the surface of the eye. Nevertheless, it is a point that is useful for all diseases of the eye, including glaucoma and central retinitis.

Sometimes, when I needle Yanagiya's GB-20 on patients who have *katakori*, they tell me it feels like this point is the very center of the tension. It is possible for a patient to feel stiffness around GB-21 when the problem is actually in the occipital area, which is seen in cases of occipital neuralgia.

TB-20 *(kaku-son / jiǎo sūn)*   ★

(SYSTEMATIC): "Above the auricle, at the center. There is a depression when the mouth is opened."

(ACUPUNCTURE): Located on the temporal area next to the uppermost point of the auricle [that is, the superior auricular point]."

(ILLUSTRATED): "Fold the ear forward, and locate the point on the hairline next to the top corner of the folded ear. Pressing this point and opening the mouth cause a depression to form by the contraction of the temporal muscle. This depression disappears when the mouth is closed."

LOCATION: Fold the ear forward, and locate the point on the scalp 0.3 unit above the hairline next to the top of the ear (Fig. 2-10).

PALPATION: Mark a provisional point on the temporal area next to the top of the ear. Fibers of the temporalis can be palpated by pressing and moving the finger ver-

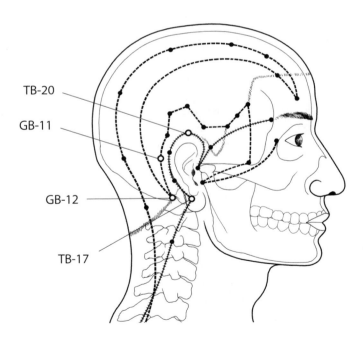

Fig. 2-10

tically back and forth over the point. Find the point that is tender. When the mouth is opened, the muscle moves to create a depression. However, do not use this to locate the point; rather, determine the site of the reaction.

INSERTION: Use a diagonal, superficial insertion with the tip of the needle pointed toward the eye.

INDICATION: TB-20 is effective for tinnitus, but it is best not to insert the needle more than a few millimeters or to produce a needle sensation, as these can make the tinnitus worse. Apply direct moxibustion for cataracts.

TB-17 (*ei-fū / yì fēng*)

(SYSTEMATIC): "In the depression behind the ear."

LOCATION: In the depression between the mandible and the mastoid process (Fig. 2-10).

PALPATION: Place the middle (or index) finger in the notch between the mandible and the mastoid process and work it superiorly, moving it vertically back and forth. When there is no reaction (or induration) in the depression, this point is not indicated; it is indicated only when there is an induration. When a patient has Mèniére's disease or a similar disorder, an induration can be found at TB-17. Thus, this point has diagnostic value. To examine these points for the purpose of diagnosis, stand at the head of the table with the patient supine and palpate both sides at the same time with your middle fingers. However, for treatment purposes, having the patient in the side-lying position is more advantageous.

INSERTION: With the patient in the side-lying position and the indicated side up, insert a needle shallowly in one of two ways:

- Vertically
- Diagonally, anteriorly, and superiorly.

A needle sensation in the ear is beneficial in cases of ear disease. In cases of tinnitus, however, a strong needle sensation must be avoided because it can worsen the ringing in the ear. Three cones of thread-like moxa can also be applied in addition to needling.

INDICATION: TB-17 is effective for all ear diseases including tinnitus, loss of hearing, and otitis media. It is also useful for stubborn cases of dizziness and paralysis of the facial nerve. Also, because the parotid gland underlies this point, it is obviously used for parotitis. And since it is close to the throat, it can be used for pain and discomfort in the throat as well as coughing due to throat problems.

GB-11 (*atama-kyō-in / tóu qiào yīn*)

(*SYSTEMATIC*): "Above the mastoid process and below the occipital bone. Movement can be felt in the hand."

(*CLARIFICATION*): "Movement refers to [pulsation of] an artery. This is why it is stated, 'can be felt in the hand'."

(*OKABE, 1974*): "One-and-a-half units posterior to the center of the auricle. Locate in the cranial suture."

LOCATION: Fold the top of the ear down, and locate the point on the scalp next to the posterior corner of the ear. It is 0.2 unit posterior to the hairline (Fig. 2-10).

PALPATION: Pressing the point posterior to the ear just inside the hairline, and moving the finger back and forth, you can feel the fibers of the occipitofrontal muscle. Find the most tender point either on the muscle or in the depression. When the reaction is not clear, palpate above and below the area.

INSERTION: With the patient in the side-lying position and the indicated point up, use a superficial insertion and retain the needle. The needle may point superiorly or inferiorly.

INDICATION: GB-11 is effective for tinnitus. Do not use strong stimulation when selecting it for this purpose; excessive stimulation sometimes aggravates the ringing in the ears.

GB-12 (*kan-kotsu / wán gǔ*)

(*SYSTEMATIC*): "Behind the ear; four-tenths of a unit behind the hairline."

(*ACUPUNCTURE*): "Palpate the posterior border of the mastoid process from the tip superiorly. You quickly reach a slight depression. This is the inferior mastoid notch. Locate this point where there is a strong penetrating sensation when the inferior mastoid notch is pressed."

LOCATION: There are two locations for GB-12:

- *Location A.* At the inferior margin of the mastoid process, just posterior to the insertion of the sternocleidomastoid muscle (Fig. 2-10).
- *Location B.* Higher up, in the depression on its posterior border (Fig. 2-11).

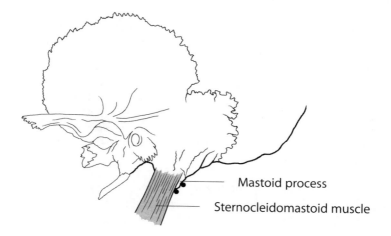

Mastoid process

Sternocleidomastoid muscle

Fig. 2-11

PALPATION: This depends on its location:

- *Location A.* Press the tip of the mastoid process (insertion of sternocleidomastoid muscle) with the tip of the middle finger, and move it back and forth. Next, press the posterior tip of the mastoid process firmly to find the most tender point.
- *Location B.* Palpate upward along the bone from the tip of the mastoid process to the first small depression. Press the middle finger superiorly toward the bone while making small rotations. You can also press with the tip of the thumb, bending it at the distal joint. Going further up on the posterior border of the mastoid process, you come to Yanagiya's GB-20.

INSERTION: Both locations can be needled with the patient lying face down, but it is even better to have the patient on their side. Insert needle to a depth of 0.2 to 0.5 unit.

- *Location A.* Aim the tip of the needle anteriorly and superiorly, toward the opening of the ear.
- *Location B.* Aim the tip of the needle either anteriorly or anteriorly and superiorly.

INDICATION: Retain the needle in GB-12 for insomnia. This point is also good for ear problems, headaches, *katakori* (see discussion at points ST-12 and GB-21) and discomfort in the occipital area. In some cases, these symptoms are not resolved until GB-12 is treated.

DISCUSSION: In *Guide to Secret One-Needle Technique,* GB-12 is featured as follows under the heading "No. 5, the Point for Pain in the Ear" (Fig. 2-12):

> The posterior tip of the mastoid process; the insertion of the sternocleidomastoid muscle. When the head is slightly extended, there is a slight depression where the sternocleidomastoid muscle attaches to the mastoid process. The direction of insertion should be toward the opening of the ear. Insert slowly and go under the inferior and medial aspect of the mastoid process. When a needle sensation is felt in the ear, withdraw the needle slightly. If there is no sensation [in the ear], withdraw the needle and reinsert. (Yanagiya, 1955)

An effective approach to symptomatic treatment is to produce a mild needle sensation in the area that is giving the patient the most trouble. In the case of ear problems, of course, the sensation should be inside the ear. Once you become proficient, this sensation can be produced almost without fail, but this is not so easy for beginners. In order to produce a needle sensation, you can either needle a recommended point like GB-12, or palpate around the problem area to locate the most tender or indurated point.

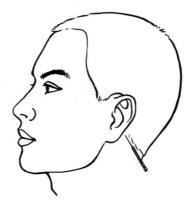

Fig. 2-12

BL-2 (*san-chiku / zǎn zhú*)

(SYSTEMATIC): "In the depression at the head of the eyebrow, otherwise known as the root of the eyebrow."

(ILLUSTRATED): "Above the inner canthus, on the medial end of the eyebrow. Probing will reveal a depression (indentation). By pressing with a fingernail and moving it back and forth, one can feel a lumpy strand that is the supraorbital nerve. Strong pressure causes a strong but pleasant sensation throughout the frontal region. Locate the point here."

LOCATION: In the depression at the medial end of the eyebrow. Tender points can be found in three places (Fig. 2-13):

- *Location A.* In the flat depression at the medial end of the eyebrow.
- *Location B.* On the border of the medial superior angle of the orbit.
- *Location C.* Between locations A and B.

PALPATION: There are three different ways of palpating this point:

- *Location A.* Press the medial end of the eyebrow in a medial and superior direction.
- *Location B.* Press the medial superior angle of the orbit with the index or middle finger, and move it back and forth, as if working the finger between the eyeball and the socket.

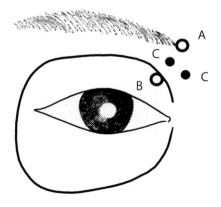

Fig. 2-13

37

- *Location C.* Press medially with the fingertip, applying small rotations.

I tend to use location C the most, followed by locations B and A. Locations B and C differ from the standard location given in textbooks.

INSERTION: For locations A and C, the needle should be pointed medially, and inserted 0.1 or 0.2 unit. Then apply rotations of small amplitude and retain the needle.

At location B, the needle is pointed in the direction of the eye socket. While inserting the needle, gently press the eyeball downward with the middle, ring, and little fingers of the supporting hand. Actually, very little pressure need be applied on the eye. It is as if you were resting your fingers on it. The depth of the needle is just enough to feel the arrival of qi. This is generally about a third of a unit, but sometimes I go as deep as half a unit.

When you needle location B, you may cause bleeding or a black eye. Therefore, use the thinnest needle possible and try to get results with superficial insertion. Bleeding at locations A and C, on the other hand, is actually to be welcomed. If the point shows signs of bleeding, press the point and squeeze out a drop or two of blood. Sometimes I even use a three-edged needle to draw a few drops of blood from these points. Nevertheless, too much pressing and squeezing of these points can cause internal bleeding in those with congestion in their face or delicate blood vessels. That is why one must be precise and practiced in bleeding these points.

INDICATION: These vary, depending on the location:

- *Location A.* Facial neuralgia, facial paralysis.
- *Location B.* Eye strain.
- *Location C.* Facial neuralgia, eye strain, congestion due to eye disease, congestion in eyes (bloodshot eyes), diminished visual acuity.

DISCUSSION: In the facial area, points around the orbit and those above the zygomatic process are especially prone to bleeding, so special care must be taken in needling them. If it is a point that is hidden by clothing, one can calmly tell the patient that the bruise will go away in several days, but a black eye or a bruise on the face is hard to hide. This is especially problematic for women. Back when Chinese needles were popular, I did a vertical insertion in ST-1 on my elder sister. There was some bleeding and bruising after I removed the needle, and I was at a loss about what to do. It was distressing because she could not open her eye fully, and it took a couple of weeks for the black eye to go away. Just thinking about this incident still upsets me. To avoid such accidents, there is the alternative strategy of using distal points to treat the eyes. Yanagiya's GB-20 is actually much more effective for eye strain, diminished eyesight, and some eye diseases. Some patients who are aware of this tell me they like the point on the back (Yanagiya's GB-20) better than the one on the face (BL-2).

BL-1 *(sei-mei / jīng míng)*   ★

(SYSTEMATIC): "Just medial to the inner canthus."

(ILLUSTRATED): "In the depression, one-tenth of a unit medial to the inner canthus."

LOCATION: In the depression medial to the inner canthus (Fig. 2-14).

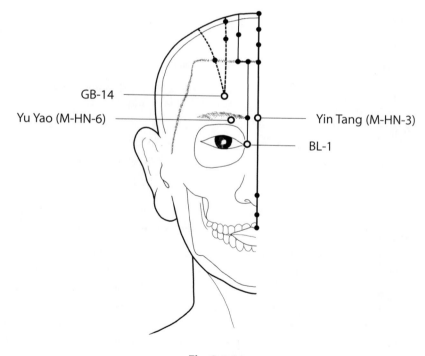

GB-14

Yu Yao (M-HN-6)

Yin Tang (M-HN-3)

BL-1

Fig. 2-14

PALPATION: Pressing the medial aspect of the inner canthus, one finds a depression and ridge just next to the nasal bone. Stick the fingertip in this depression, as if pressing a nail into the deepest part (location A). Sometimes there is tenderness on the ridge (location B). The points I use most often are on either side of location B, which I shall call location C. These are the openings of the tear ducts (Fig. 2-15).

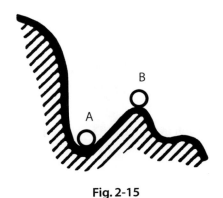

Fig. 2-15

INSERTION: These vary according to their location:

- *Location A.* Insert 0.1 unit in the depression, with the tip pointed medially.
- *Location B.* Insert 0.1 unit vertically on the ridge. Apply a little rotation.
- *Location C (either side of B).* Use a 40mm, No. 0 needle to penetrate the tear duct. When there is pain from dacryocystitis (inflammation of the lacrimal glands), it is soothing to lightly prick or stroke the opening with the needle tip.

INDICATION: Again, these vary according to their location:

- *Locations A and B.* Facial neuralgia, pain from eye strain.
- *Location C.* Problems with lacrimation, especially when there is pain.

DISCUSSION: There used to be an old woman in my neighborhood who was skilled at removing irritants from the eyes. She used to come by from time to time to sort through the needles I was going to discard. She would take the 50mm, No. 3 to 5 needles and wrap paper around the body of each needle so that only the tip protruded. She used this device to scrape and remove dust and small debris from the cornea. This woman could clean out small irritants in peoples' eyes that the local ophthalmologist could do nothing to alleviate.

This kind of folk remedy was not considered unusual where I come from. My own mother used hot needles to pierce skin eruptions. She would take a fairly thick needle and get the tip red hot, then stick it into the middle of the boil. This was an application of the 'fire needle' technique. I never actually observed her doing these treatments, but she told me people used to request it. These are interesting examples that suggest how widely needles were employed in the past as a part of folk medicine.

LI-20 (gei-gō / yíng xiāng)   ★

(SYSTEMATIC): "Above LI-19, below the nose, next to the hole."

(ILLUSTRATED): "On the upper end of the nasolabial groove. Located half a unit lateral to the nasal opening."

(ACUPUNCTURE): "It is at the level of the ala nasi in the nasolabial groove. The place where the ala nasi protrudes the farthest is called the ala nasi point. A penetrating sensation is felt in the nose and upper teeth when this point is pressed with the fingertip at the level of the ala nasi in the nasolabial groove (which forms when a person laughs). Locate the point here."

LOCATION: In the nasolabial groove at the level of the ala nasi, or next to the bottom of the nasal opening (Fig. 2-16).

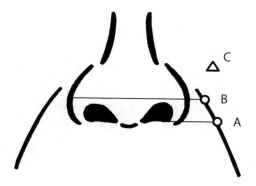

Fig. 2-16

PALPATION: Using the index or middle finger, probe the upper end of the nasolabial groove. Tenderness often appears slightly lateral to the nasolabial groove. There is actually another point at the level of the top of the ala nasi, about one finger-width lateral to the point (location C). Tenderness can be found by moving the fingertip back and forth diagonally over this point.

INSERTION: Insert the needle diagonally and superiorly. The insertion depth can be quite deep (up to 1cm).

INDICATION: Nasal diseases, such as nasal discharge, nasal congestion, sneezing, and loss of sense of smell; ear problems, such as a sense of blockage and loss of hearing.

M-HN-3 *(yin-dō / yìn táng)* ★

(XU, 1439): "In the center, between the eyebrows."

(YANG, 1601): "In the depression."

(YANAGIYA, 1955): "Stroke the patient with a fingertip three times between the eyebrows down from GV-24 to the bridge of the nose. Feel for depressions and protrusions in the cranium beneath the skin. A protrusion can be felt on both sides just before the fingertip comes between the eyebrows. The fingertip comes into a V-shaped groove at the bottom end of the space between the eyebrows. Just before the fingertip goes down over the bottom of the V, there is a slight depression. Use this point. It is the miscellaneous point M-HN-3."

LOCATION: In the depression between the eyebrows (Fig. 2-14).

PALPATION: A groove can be found when stroking down between the eyebrows and going down onto the bridge of the nose. Use the tip of your index or middle finger to stroke vertically and confirm the location of this groove. Once you find it, shake the fingertip horizontally to look for tenderness. Move the fingertip back and forth horizontally as you work your way downward in the groove.

INSERTION: Insert a 40mm, No. 0 or 00 needle, and aim the tip downward as far as it will go. When it runs into the (nasal) bone, withdraw it slightly. It is good when a needle sensation is felt in the nose (Fig. 2-17).

INDICATION: Sinus and nasal diseases.

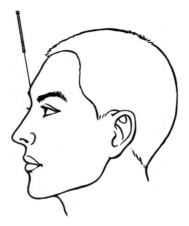

Fig. 2-17

DISCUSSION: Sinusitis begins with sneezing and nasal discharge. In serious cases there is such a large amount of copious discharge that the patient wonders where all the fluid could possibly come from. In cases of allergic rhinitis, the area around the eyes begins to itch, and the nasal discharge is accompanied by tearing. This is known in Japanese as *mejiru-hanajiru* (literally 'eye juice–nose juice'). In some cases, rhinitis can cause thick nasal discharge, nasal congestion, and frontal headaches. I experienced this condition last winter. Points such as M-HN-3, LI-20, BL-2, GV-22, and GV-23 became tender, but M-HN-3 was particularly tender. When a point is extremely tender, it feels good to have it needled, and one would like to have the needle left in forever. It may be acceptable to treat local points in this way, but it is much more effective, after all, to regulate the meridians that are at the root of the condition.

Nasal discharge, tearing, and sputum are all related to fluids. This brings to mind a passage in Chapter 10 of *Vital Axis*. Under the section dealing with the symptoms of the Large Intestine meridian it says: "When that which controls the thin fluids *(shin/jīn)* gives rise to disease." Some of the main symptoms related to the Large Intestine meridian may be regarded as conditions related to the thin fluids. The Small Intestine meridian is said to control the thick fluids *(eki/yè)*. Among the yin meridians, the Lung, Spleen, and Kidney are associated with fluids. In my own case, treating the Kidney and Large Intestine meridians cleared up my condition. I used KI-10, the sea (water) point, and LI-2, the spring (water) point.[2]

GB-14 *(yō-haku / yáng bái)*

(SYSTEMATIC): "One unit above the eyebrow; straight above the pupil."

(ILLUSTRATED): "One unit above the center of the eyebrow. Probing with the finger, one detects a depression in the bone. Pressing strongly there is a sensation that penetrates into the head. Locate the point here."

(ACUPUNCTURE): "It is on the vertical line that goes through the pupil when looking straight ahead. Pressing with the fingertip two centimeters above the upper margin of the eyebrow, one finds the rise of the superciliary arch. GB-14 is located just above this rise."

LOCATION: In a depression, one finger-width above and just slightly lateral to the center of the eyebrow (Fig. 2-14).

PALPATION: There is a ridge in the bone one finger-width above the center of the eyebrow. There is a depression just lateral to this. Pressing this region with the tip of the middle finger, and moving it back and forth horizontally, you will feel something like a fiber inside the depression. This is the frontal nerve. It is especially easy to palpate when it is inflamed.

INSERTION: Insert a 40mm, No. 0 or 00 needle, and point the tip inferiorly or superiorly. The depth should be between 0.2 to 0.3 unit. The insertion must not be painful.

INDICATION: Trigeminal neuralgia (of the supraorbital nerve). For acute and/or intense pain, treat the opposite (unaffected) side. Other indications include eye strain and discomfort in the eyes when watching television, frontal headaches, and drooping eyelids from facial paralysis.

M-HN-6 *(gyo-yō / yú yāo)*

(YANG, 1601): "In the midpoint of the eyebrow."

(YAMASHITA, 1972): "This point is on the middle of the eyebrow."

LOCATION: Slightly medial to the midpoint of the eyebrow. It lies in the supraorbital foramen (Fig. 2-14).

PALPATION: Dragging the fingertip laterally over the eyebrow from BL-2, you will run across a depression. Stand your index finger on end and move it back and forth horizontally in the depression. You can feel something like a fiber in the depression that is tender.

INSERTION: Insert the needle diagonally and superiorly. The needle will go very deep if the supraorbital foramen is penetrated, but keep the needle depth shallow.

INDICATION: Neuralgia of the supraorbital nerve, eye strain and fatigue in the eyes from too much reading or watching television.

ST-2 (*shi-haku / sì bái*)

(SYSTEMATIC): "One unit below the eye. On the cheek bone in the hollow [in front] of the zygomatic bone."

(ILLUSTRATED): "One unit below the lower border of the orbit. Pressing the area below the orbit on the surface, one can feel some tissue or muscle that runs from the inner canthus to the lower end of the zygomatic bone. [The point is] on the upper margin of this muscle and directly below the pupil. Locate it where there is a slight depression in the bone."

LOCATION: One finger-width below the lower border of the orbit in the depression (Fig. 2-18).

PALPATION: Placing the tip of a finger at the midpoint of the lower margin of the orbit and pressing as you move it back and forth slightly will reveal a tender point, which is ST-1. Dragging the finger straight down, it falls into a depression. Locate ST-2 by pressing and rotating the fingertip inside the upper end of this depression to find the tender point.

INSERTION: Use a vertical, shallow insertion.

INDICATION: Facial paralysis, paralysis of the oculomotor nerve.

ST-4 (*chi-sō / dì cāng*)

(ELABORATION): "Four-tenths of a unit from the corner of the lips on both sides."

45

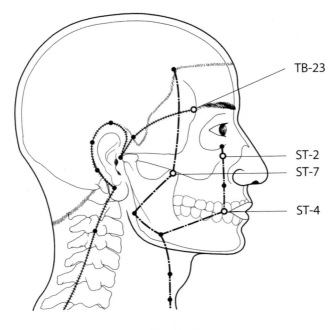

TB-23

ST-2
ST-7

ST-4

Fig. 2-18

(*ILLUSTRATED*): "Four-tenths of a unit lateral to the corner of the mouth."

LOCATION: Just lateral to the corner of the mouth and medial to the nasolabial groove, where sometimes one can feel a pulsation (Fig. 2-18).

PALPATION: When the pulsation is unclear, locate the point at the midpoint between the corner of the mouth and nasolabial groove.

INSERTION: Use a superficial insertion.

INDICATION: For facial paralysis when the obicularis oris muscle is paralyzed and the patient cannot pucker the lips, apply three cones of thread-like moxa.

ST-7 (*ge-kan / xià guān*)

(*SYSTEMATIC*): "Below GB-3, on the inferior margin in the hollow beneath the pulsation in front of the ear. There is a hole when the mouth is closed. When the mouth is opened wide, the hole closes."

(*ILLUSTRATED*): "On the inferior border of the zygomatic arch in the depression anterior to the mandibular condyle. It is approximately two finger-widths anterior to the ear; under the zygomatic arch in the depression anterior to the mandibular condyle. When the mouth is opened, the condylar process moves forward and [the hole] closes."

LOCATION: On the inferior border of the zygomatic arch, just below GB-3 (Fig. 2-18).

PALPATION: Tracing the middle finger along the bottom of the zygomatic arch, starting from just in front of the ear, you can feel the muscle fibers running vertically. The point is tender.

INSERTION: Use a vertical, shallow (up to 5mm into the muscle) insertion. For temporomandibular joint (TMJ) problems with spontaneous pain, an intradermal needle can be retained instead.

INDICATION: Pain in the TMJ when the mouth is opened, and also when pain accompanies biting down.

TB-23 (*shi-chiku-kū / sī zhú kōng*) ★

(*SYSTEMATIC*): "Posterior to the eyebrow, inside the depression."

(*ILLUSTRATED*): "It is a little medial to the lateral end of the eyebrow where there is a slight depression in the bone. Pressing this point firmly, there will be a deep and penetrating sensation."

LOCATION: In the depression slightly medial to the lateral end of the eyebrow (Fig. 2-18).

PALPATION: Placing the fingertip vertically on the point and moving it back and forth horizontally will make the depression obvious.

INSERTION: Use a superficial insertion.

INDICATION: Facial paralysis.

GB-1 (*dō-ji-ryō / tóng zǐ liáo*) ★

(*SYSTEMATIC*): "Lateral to the eye, half a unit from the [outer] canthus."

(ILLUSTRATED): "On the bone, half a unit lateral to the outer canthus. Probing a little with the fingertip will reveal a slight depression in the bone."

LOCATION: On the lateral border of the orbit (Fig. 2-19).

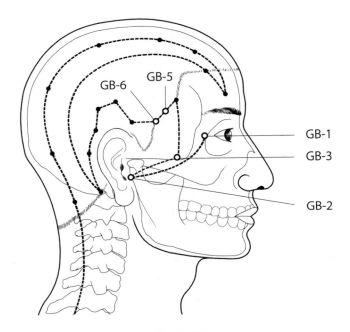

Fig. 2-19

PALPATION: There are three possible points (Fig. 2-20):

- *Location A.* Work the fingertip toward the border of the orbit from the side, and select the most tender point.
- *Location B.* There is a slight depression in the lateral border of the orbit. Locate this by moving the fingertip up and down as well as sideways.
- *Location C.* Seek the most tender point in the muscle lateral to the orbit.

INSERTION: Use superficial insertions, but vary your technique according to the location:

- *Location A.* Insert the needle shallowly (5mm) toward the eye.
- *Location B.* Just break the skin (superficial).
- *Location C.* Aim the needle toward the eye (superficial).

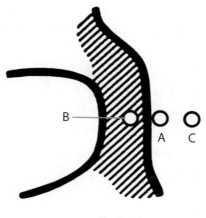

Fig. 2-20

Locations A and C tend to bleed easily, so avoid any veins that are visible on the surface.

INDICATION: Eye diseases, especially those affecting the surface, and injuries to the eye on the lateral aspect.

GB-2 (*chō-e / tīng huì*)

(*SYSTEMATIC*): "In the depression just in front of the ear. [It is] found when the mouth is opened wide. [It is] where a pulsation can be palpated."

(*ACUPUNCTURE*): "The tragus protrudes over the opening of the ear, and the notch below it is known as the intertragic notch. Locate [this point] in the depression just anterior to the intertragic notch."

LOCATION: Anterior to the auditory meatus, on the border of the mandible (Fig. 2-19).

PALPATION: Placing a finger just in front of the opening of the ear, open the mouth a little so that a depression forms in front of the tragus. Stroke the posterior border of the mandible from top to bottom with the fingertip, and you will find a place where the finger catches and which is painful when pressed. Often you will find a little nodule shaped like a grain of rice that is not very hard. Sometimes this reaction appears above at SI-19, but after examining many patients, I find that the reaction appears more often on the lower end. Sometimes it appears lower than the intertragic notch.

INSERTION: Use a vertical, superficial insertion. It is easier to insert the needle when the mouth is slightly open. However, when the little nodule is the target, the mouth can stay closed. In either case, the mouth should remain closed while retaining the needle.

INDICATION: Jaw pain and ear problems, such as tinnitus.

GB-3 (jō-kan / shàng guān)

(SYSTEMATIC): "The upper margin of the anterior ear, on the border of the zygomatic bone. Opening the mouth, a hole appears."

(ILLUSTRATED): "On the superior border of the zygomatic bone, slightly posterior to the anterior hairline of the sideburns. Strong pressure here is painful."

(OKABE, 1974): "On the upper border of the midpoint of the zygomatic arch. There is a depression when the mouth is opened."

LOCATION: On the superior border of the zygomatic bone, on the margin of the hairline (Fig. 2-19).

PALPATION: Trace the upper border of the zygomatic arch with a fingertip from front to back to reach the hairline. Applying pressure as you move back and forth horizontally, you will feel muscle fibers. Locate the most painful point. Sometimes it is 0.2 to 0.3 unit behind the hairline.

INSERTION: Insert a needle diagonally and downward 0.3 to 0.5 unit along the inside of the zygomatic arch.

INDICATION: Tooth pain, facial neuralgia.

GB-5 (ken-ro / xuán lú)

(SYSTEMATIC): "In the center of the temples."

(ILLUSTRATED): "In the temporal area on the posterior end of the hairline on the temple. One unit below GB-4. It is in the temporalis muscle where movement in the muscle can be felt when biting down."

LOCATION: The point is located about one unit anterior and superior to GB-6 (Fig. 2-19).

PALPATION: First locate GB-6. Rotate the tip of the middle finger in the temporal area at the level of the eyebrow to feel the fibers of the temporalis muscle. The tight or tender point on the posterior margin of the temporalis muscle is GB-6. Then move the finger one unit anterior and superior to GB-6. Locate the hardest point by making small circles with your fingertip. This is GB-5.

INSERTION: Use a vertical or diagonal insertion toward the feet to a depth of about 3mm. Be careful because this area bleeds easily. Actually, you may want to bleed this point a little when it is very hard, or there is circulatory congestion in the head.

INDICATION: Temporal headache, migraine, trigeminal neuralgia, tooth pain.

GB-6 (ken-ri / xuán lí)   ★★

(SYSTEMATIC): "On the lower margin of the temples."

(OKABE, 1974): "On the lateral hairline of the head at the level of the upper margin of the eyebrow."

LOCATION: In the temporalis muscle at the level of the eyebrow, one unit below GB-5 (Fig. 2-19).

PALPATION: Rotate the tip of the middle finger in the temporal area at the level of the eyebrow to feel the fibers of the temporalis muscle. The tight or tender point on the posterior margin of the temporalis muscle is GB-6.

INSERTION & INDICATION: Same as those described for GB-5.

DISCUSSION: Compare the reactions at GB-5 and GB-6, and select the point at which the reaction is more pronounced. Often temporal headaches can be relieved just by treating points of the Gallbladder meridian on the leg. In very chronic cases, however, points on the temple must be needled to get results.

POINTS ON THE
NECK AND SHOULDERS

ST-9 (*jin-gei / rén yíng*)

(SYSTEMATIC): "The great pulse on the neck. [It is] where a pulsation can be palpated. It is on either side of the laryngeal prominence. [It is] used to examine the qi in the five yin organs."

(ILLUSTRATED): "On the anterior aspect of the neck one-and-a-half units lateral to the laryngeal prominence. It is over the pulsation of the common carotid artery."

LOCATION: Where the pulsation of the common carotid artery is strongest (Fig. 2-21).

PALPATION: Place the tip of your middle finger on the point where you feel the strongest pulsation, and move it back and forth to find a tiny groove, which is the bifurcation of the carotid artery. If it is difficult to locate, pinch the skin in the area above the artery, and insert the needle in the point where the skin is thickest. I use this method of locating ST-9 when I retain an intradermal needle.

INSERTION: Use a vertical, shallow insertion up to the wall of the carotid artery. This is a very sensitive point, so simple insertion and gentle manipulation with a thin needle works best.

INDICATION: Sore throat, hoarseness, or sensation of something stuck in the throat. An intradermal needle can be used on one side for pain or discomfort in the throat.

DISCUSSION: ST-9 lies directly over the common carotid artery and close to the carotid sinus, which has baroreceptors related to changes in blood pressure. Shirota Bunshi, a student of Sawada Ken, developed a direct insertion technique for the treatment of high blood pressure, asthma, and chronic pain conditions such as

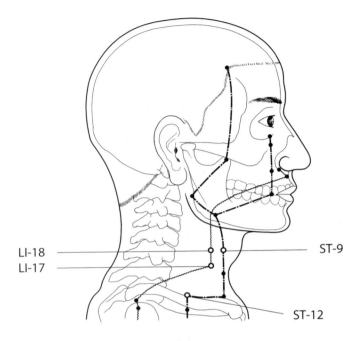

Fig. 2-21

arthritis. In this technique, a needle is inserted until it runs into the wall of the carotid artery. The needle is retained, and the head of the needle moves back and forth with the pulsation of the artery. I do not use ST-9 in this way and do not retain the needle.

ST-9 is known as *jingei/rén yíng*, and taking the pulse here at the carotid artery seems to predate the pulse diagnosis at the radial artery, which is the common practice today. The term *jingei*—pulse diagnosis—refers to a comparison of the carotid pulse with the radial one, and is mentioned in both *Basic Questions* and *Vital Axis*. In Japan, Dōkei Ogura revived this method in the 1950s and has been successfully applying *jingei* pulse diagnosis in his practice. Ogura palpates the pulses with the patient seated. He uses the thumb and index finger of one hand to palpate the carotid artery on both sides, and palpates the radial artery with the index, middle, and ring fingers of his other hand. I have never used this technique in my practice, but it shows that there are a number of different approaches to pulse diagnosis that can be applied successfully in acupuncture.

LI-17 *(ten-tei / tiān dǐng)*   ★★★

(SYSTEMATIC): "Above ST-12 in line with LI-18. One-and-a-half units posterior to ST-11."

(ILLUSTRATED): "The artery on either side of the laryngeal prominence is ST-9, and just lateral to this point is LI-18. [From this point] go down over the sternocleidomastoid muscle; it is one unit inferior on the posterior aspect of the sternocleidomastoid muscle."

LOCATION: I locate this point about three finger-widths above ST-12. It is just above the posterior margin of the sternocleidomastoid muscle (Fig. 2-21).

PALPATION: Bend your thumb at the first joint to form a hook, then press the point with the tip of your thumb. Press and work your way down from LI-18 until you feel a projection of the spine. This point is where the tenderness is greatest and where pressing causes a radiating sensation in the shoulder and arm.

INSERTION: Needle with the patient in the seated position. Carefully insert a 30mm, No. 01 or 02 needle, angled posteriorly. Insert slowly as you rotate the needle. When the tip of the needle reaches the surface of the induration, there is a pleasant needle sensation that extends to the GB-20 area, the upper arm, the interscapualr area, the pectoral region, the ear, or the throat. Be sure to avoid deep insertion and the use of thick needles at this point.

Ask the patient about the needle sensation, and feel the hardness of the tissue around the point with your fingers as you slowly insert the needle. Then it is up to you whether you insert the needle a little deeper into the center of the induration, or stop on the surface of the induration. As long as you do not intend to force the needle in, you will make the right choice. If it is the first treatment, play it safe and retain the needle with the tip right on the surface of the induration. In time, the point will soften up so that the needle will go in deeper by itself.

INDICATION: The point is good for *katakori* (see discussion under ST-12 and GB-21), especially when it is related to ear or throat problems. It is also good for tension in the interscapular area, thoracic outlet syndrome, and numbness in the hand, as well as for a feeling of obstruction in the throat.

ST-12 *(ketsu-bon / quē pén)*

(SYSTEMATIC): "In the depression behind the clavicle."

(ILLUSTRATED): "On the midclavicular line in the supraclavicular fossa. Probing in this area, one finds string-like tender tissue."

LOCATION: On the pulsation in the supraclavicular fossa (Fig. 2-21).

PALPATION: Moving a fingertip lightly back and forth in the supraclavicular fossa, you will find muscle fibers running vertically. The point is close to where a pulsation can be felt with light pressure. Look for the hardest point. Exerting pressure that is too strong can cause numbness or discomfort in the arm.

INSERTION: As with LI-17, needle this point carefully with the thinnest needle. Once there is a mild and pleasant sensation in the upper arm or interscapular area, the right depth has been reached. I usually treat points in the supraclavicular fossa with the patient in a seated position, but one has to be careful about pneumothorax and needle shock. Just remember to avoid thick needles, deep insertion, and strong manipulation. These points are not for those practitioners who believe that the deeper the insertion and the stronger the stimulation, the better.

INDICATION: *Katakori*, numbness in the arms, pain in the upper back, abnormalities in the viscera.

DISCUSSION: *Katakori* (neck and shoulder stiffness) is a troublesome symptom. When I had pleuritis in my youth, and again recently, I experienced strong *katakori*. It is well known that the adhesions that result from pleuritis can cause terrible *katakori*. I remember receiving acupuncture at points like BL-17 and BL-43, SI-11, PC-4, GB-21, GB-34, and GB-41, and will also never forget how painful it was to receive moxibustion at GB-21. As for the more recent episode of *katakori*, I am not sure what caused it. I attempted some symptomatic points on myself, looking for the focal point of tension, but I couldn't seem to get at it. So I had about ten young acupuncturists from my study group try their hands. None of them were able to hit the bull's eye. The more they missed, the worse the *katakori* seemed to get, and I became more and more irritated.

The stiffness seemed to be concentrated under GB-21, and I decided to needle myself once more. After attempting various points, I finally discovered how to get the needle tip on just the right point. It moved around, but was somewhere between ST-12 and LI-17, on the side of the neck. I felt the needle sensation under GB-21, between the scapulae, and even in the center of my head. My *katakori* must have been caused by some abnormality in the cervical vertebrae or the scalene muscles. Anyway, the secret to needling such points is to locate the tightest or hardest point, and get the needle tip right on it.

For the final step in treating patients with *katakori*, I have them sit on the side of the table and stand behind them. I place my hands on their shoulders, with the four fingers in front and the thumbs on the back. Then I palpate both sides at once with a scraping motion from ST-12 to GB-21. It is easy to find the most indurated points this way. It is said that the Japanese are especially prone to *katakori*, and I find that people with rounded shoulders or hunched backs tend to have it. Active points also tend to show up in the supraclavicular fossa in such patients.

GB-21 (*ken-sei / jiān jǐng*)   ★★★

(*SYSTEMATIC*): "In the depression on the shoulder, above ST-12, in front of the big bone."

(*ILLUSTRATED*): "On the anterior margin of the trapezius and in line with the midclavicular line. In other words, it is directly above ST-12. Strong pressure here causes pain. It has been said from the olden days that when the second, third, and fourth fingers are placed on top of the shoulder, GB-21 is under the third finger."

(*ACUPUNCTURE*): "In the midpoint between the spinous process of the seventh cervical vertebra and the tip of the acromion. Locate this point where pressing on the trapezius causes a sensation to radiate to the anterior neck."

LOCATION: On the anterior margin of the trapezius, slightly anterior to the midpoint between the spinous process of the seventh cervical vertebra and the tip of the acromion. It is where the strap of a backpack comes across the shoulder, and it is under the middle finger when three fingers are placed over this area (Fig. 2-22).

PALPATION: Start from LI-16 on the lateral end of the shoulder and lightly press toward the neck with the middle finger. You will find an induration at approximately the midclavicular line. Actually, the location varies between patients and over time. Often it appears in a more anterior direction, closer to ST-12. Pinch the point with your thumb and three fingers and the patient will say "That's it!" This is, however, not quite the same location as when you press. Use the point that is the most reactive.

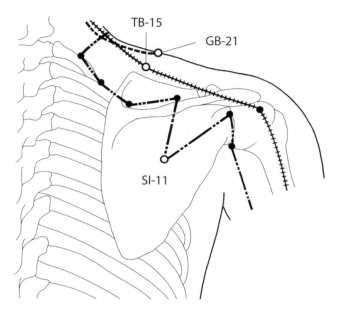

TB-15

GB-21

SI-11

Fig. 2-22

INSERTION: Stand on the left side of the patient, who is lying face down, and insert the needle vertically. In this position, the needle can go quite deeply. When a 40mm needle goes in about halfway, the needle should come up against an induration and you should feel a gummy resistance at the needletip. It is not good when the needle goes in and out without any resistance. Should that happen, reinsert the needle or change the direction of the needle after withdrawing it to just under the skin. Imagine that you are trying to pinpoint an acupuncture point that is floating in midair. Withdraw, reinsert, and apply some rotation, and eventually you will hit the mark. When you do, the needle sensation goes to the occipital area, ear, eye, throat, and temples, and otherwise down to the interscapular area, the pectoral area, and even to the abdomen. Basically, the sensation travels to wherever the patient feels the tension.

When the patient is in a seated position, I insert the needle vertically and superficially. In this position, shallow needling is enough to produce a needle sensation. This is a technique I use at the end of a treatment. Another good technique for this position comes from Yanagiya's text, *Guide to Secret One-Needle Technique*, that is, the trapezius is pinched up between the thumb and four fingers, and the needle is threaded horizontally from front to back.

INDICATION: *Katakori,* headaches and toothaches, diseases above the shoulder, high blood pressure, arteriosclerosis, prevention of senility. Apply multiple cones of direct moxibustion on the affected side for toothaches or trigeminal neuralgia. When GB-21 is used for internal and gynecological problems, it relieves distention of the stomach.

DISCUSSION: When a patient has *katakori,* the sensation of stiffness will quickly subside as soon as the needle tip reaches the palpable source of the stiffness. Patients tend to experience *katakori* around the base of their neck no matter where the problem originates. Often, patients feel the stiffness around GB-21. Yet, when you palpate around the point, you find no special reaction. In this case, of course, needling the point will not do the trick. If, however, you needle points around GB-20 instead (such as Yanagiya's GB-20), sometimes a needle sensation is felt strongly in the affected area (GB-21). This is why treating *katakori* is no simple matter. Other points that work to relieve *katakori* around GB-21 include BL-15, BL-17, BL-41, BL-42, BL-43, TB-15, SI-12, and ST-12. Points like GB-20 and GB-21 are important in the treatment when a person tends toward mental stress and overuse of their arms and hands.

Classical texts emphasize the dangers of needle shock caused by needling GB-21. In *Concise Discourse on Acupuncture and Moxibustion,* Ishizaka Sōtetsu describes this phenomenon:

> It seems that unless the symptoms are severe, this point should not be needled. If the gathering vessels *(sōmyaku/zōng mài)*[3] are pierced by accident, some patients will faint. (Sōtetsu, 1812)

It is true that needle shock is very unpleasant, both for the patient and the practitioner. Ishizaka Sōkei, the son-in-law of Ishizaka Sōtetsu, explains this in more detail:

> Needle shock happens when needling causes light-headedness. Some even faint. This can happen even if an experienced acupuncturist does the needling. It is caused by severe contact with the gathering vessels. Beginners become frightened and lose their composure, and they are at a loss for what to do. (Sōkei, 1860)

This reflects my own experience. It can even make the practitioner break out in a cold sweat! Meanwhile, the patient turns white and sometimes vomits or even becomes incontinent. It is enough to make you become faint yourself. In extreme cases, one might start to think about calling an ambulance. Ishizaka Sōkei instructs as follows:

59

Do not become flustered. Quickly get a small towel or cloth and cover the nose and mouth of the person. Then firmly press the area about one unit below CV-15 with three fingers of your left hand. The patient will be revived. (Sōkei, 1860)

Once a patient of one of my teachers started feeling nauseous after being needled at ST-12, and did not seem to get better. My teacher called on a doctor in his neighborhood to help him. The doctor massaged the patient's lower abdomen for a while and the patient got better. I have adopted this method, and it has worked for me. Ishizaka Sōkei further instructs:

It is also good to needle LI-10. If the needle shock comes from needling a point on the right side, treat LI-10 on the left side. When they come around, it is also good to give them Drain the Epigastrium Decoction *(sha shin tō/xiè xīn tāng)*.[4] (Sōkei, 1860)

It is well known that needling LI-10 or ST-36 on the opposite side helps revive a patient. It is also good to have the patient drink a strong cup of tea.

TB-15 *(ten-ryō / tiān liáo)* ★★

(ZHANG, 1624): "One unit directly posterior to GB-21."

(ILLUSTRATED): "Above the superior angle of the scapula and one unit posterior to GB-21. Pressing [this point] the flesh is depressed, but in its center or to the right or left, there is a hard spot which is not bone. The point is [located right] on this spot."

LOCATION: Just above and medial to the superior angle of the scapula (Fig. 2-22).

PALPATION: Probing two finger-widths above and medial to the superior angle of the scapula, you will find a hard nodule.

INSERTION: Use a vertical, superficial insertion.

INDICATION: *Katakori* (see discussion under ST-12 and GB-21).

SI-11 *(ten-sō / tiān zōng)* ★★★

(SYSTEMATIC): "Posterior to SI-12, below the big bone in the depression."

(ILLUSTRATED): "Inferior to the midpoint of the spine of the scapula; close to the center of the infraspinous fossa. Pressing [here] there is a tender point in some muscle fibers." (Fig. 2-22)

LOCATION: Three finger-widths below the midpoint of the spine of the scapula.

PALPATION: Probing the area below the spine of the scapula, you will find muscle fibers that run vertically and diagonally in an inferior and medial direction. Press with your fingertip and move back and forth over these fibers horizontally to find a point that, when pressed, causes a penetrating pain. The patient may be seated or prone, but use light pressure because this is a sensitive point. The reaction appears within a broad area, so probe the entire infraspinous area. Sometimes, unexpectedly, it appears far below the standard location.

INSERTION: Insert diagonally in either a medial direction or superior laterally. When the needle penetrates into the fibers of the muscle, fasciculation (twitch) can cause the needle to bend if it is thin (less than No. 2). Even so, thick needles can result in too much stimulation and cause discomfort. I often use direct moxibustion instead.

INDICATION: Pain and numbness in the arm: Those who strain their arms at work often show reactions at SI-11. Other indications are problems in the shoulder joint, pectoral region and breasts, chest pain, coughing, and fever from colds.

SI-9 (*ken-tei / jiān zhēn*)

(SYSTEMATIC): "Below the acromion, posterior to LI-15 in the middle of the depression."

(ILLUSTRATED): "On the back, approximately one unit above the axillary crease. One can feel the lower margin of the glenohumoral joint by pressing with the fingers."

(ACUPUNCTURE): "Put the finger on the posterior end of the axillary crease, and move it superiorly along the muscle fibers on either side. Locate [the point] 2cm from the end of the crease." (Fig. 2-23).

LOCATION: In the midpoint between the end of the axillary crease and SI-10 (lower margin of the acromion).

PALPATION: There is a muscle that runs diagonally at the midpoint between the axillary crease and the lateral margin of the acromion (posterior fibers of the deltoid). Press with the middle finger, and move across the muscle fibers horizontally to locate the hardest point. If the reaction is found on the upper end (of the muscle), it is SI-10.

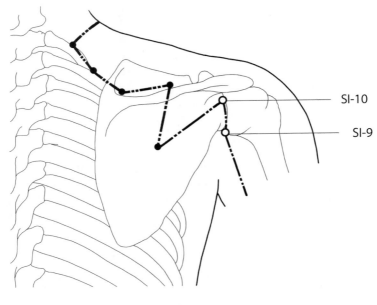

Fig. 2-23

INSERTION: Use a perpendicular insertion. The depth varies from superficial to one-third of a unit. I usually needle this point with the patient in a side-lying position, with the arm resting on the side of the body. Retain the needle in this point for patients with frozen shoulder.

INDICATION: Frozen shoulder and other shoulder joint problems.

LI-15 (*ken-gū / jiān yú*)

(SYSTEMATIC): "On the end of the shoulder, between both bones."

(ILLUSTRATED): "Two depressions form over the shoulder joint when the arm is raised. Locate [this point] in the anterior depression."

LOCATION: Between the acromion and the head of the humerus (Fig. 2-24).

PALPATION: Move the finger anteriorly from the end of the acromion and probe for tense muscle fibers. If there is any tenderness, locate the point right there; if not, locate it in the depression.

LI-15 —————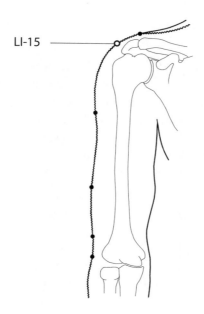

Fig. 2-24

INSERTION: When there is inflammation in the rotator cuff or the tendon of the supraspinatus muscle, insert a needle horizontally into the depression (parallel to the floor), with the patient in a seated position. The needle is thus inserted medially, up to one unit, toward the joint. When the space between the bones is small, it is hard to insert the needle very deeply. In this case, have the patient abduct the arm 90 degrees and insert the needle into the joint. When treating the patient in a side-lying position, seek a tender point close to the head of the humerus. Use a superficial insertion and retain the needle.

INDICATION: Shoulder joint problems.

GV-14 (*dai-tsui / dà zhuī*)

(SYSTEMATIC): "Above the first vertebra, in the depression."

(ILLUSTRATED): "In the space between the spinous process of the seventh cervical and first thoracic vertebrae."

LOCATION: Between the spinous process of the seventh cervical and first thoracic vertebrae (Fig. 2-25).

PALPATION: Press and move a finger back and forth between the spinous process-es to find the point. GV-14 is between the biggest protrusion at the base of the neck (C7) and the vertebra under it (T1). With the patient bending their head forward, mark the top of the seventh cervical vertebra. When the patient rights their head, the mark moves down between the vertebrae to GV-14. (If you are not sure which one is the seventh cervical vertebra, have the patient turn their head from side to side. The lowest vertebra that moves is the seventh cervical vertebra.)

INSERTION & INDICATION: Apply direct moxibustion for the early stages of a cold and upper respiratory tract infections. Multiple cones, from 15 to 50, are most effective. This method is also effective for rhinitis. For colds, contact needling, instead of moxibustion, can be applied around GV-14. When there is pathology in the cervical vertebrae and there is tenderness or pain with percussion, retain a nee-dle superficially at GV-14 or on the lateral margin of the vertebra, wherever the ten-derness or pain is clearest.

POINTS ON THE
BACK AND HIP

GV-12 (shin-chū / shēn zhù)

(SYSTEMATIC): "In the joint under the third vertebra. Locate with the patient in a prone position."

(ILLUSTRATED): "On the back, inferior to the spinous process of the third thoracic vertebra."

LOCATION: Between the spinous process of the third and fourth thoracic vertebrae (Fig. 2-25).

PALPATION: With the patient seated or prone, press the point and move the finger back and forth horizontally between the spinous processes. Reactions in the intervertebral spaces are easier to detect when the body is relaxed in the prone position. Reactions between the seventh cervical and first thoracic vertebrae are not easy to detect, but they become quite obvious below the third thoracic vertebra. The space between the spinous processes is wider, there is a marked depression, and it may feel mushy, or like a muscle or tendon instead of bone. Focus all your attention on your fingertip and practice finding these reactions.

INSERTION: Use a superficial insertion and retain the needle. Direct moxibustion is also effective.

INDICATION: Useful for upper respiratory tract infections. Also, acupuncture or moxibustion can be applied for nervous disorders when there is a reaction here.

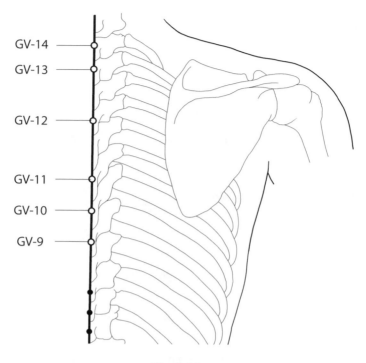

GV-14
GV-13
GV-12
GV-11
GV-10
GV-9

Fig. 2-25

GV-11 (*shin-dō / shén dào*)   ★★★

(*SYSTEMATIC*): "In the joint under the fifth vertebra. Locate with the patient in a prone position."

(*ILLUSTRATED*): "On the back, inferior to the spinous process of the fifth thoracic vertebra."

LOCATION: Between the spinous processes of the fifth and sixth thoracic vertebrae (Fig. 2-25).

PALPATION: Press the point and move the finger back and forth between the spinous processes. GV-11 is best located with the patient in a prone position; thus, the back-and-forth movement of the finger actually is in an anterior-posterior direction in relation to the practitioner. Applying light pressure as the finger moves between the spinous processes will reveal a reaction. When there is no clear reaction, make a loose fist and lightly strike the spinous processes above and below with the knuckle of your little finger. Sometimes, no tenderness or induration can be found between the vertebrae, but a reaction will instead be found on the lateral margin of the spinous process. For a more thorough search, go completely around both spinous processes.

INSERTION: Use a superficial insertion and retain the needle. Alternatively, apply direct moxibustion.

INDICATION: Nervous disorders, especially dysfunctions of the autonomic nervous system.

DISCUSSION: In Fukaya-style moxibustion, reactions between the upper thoracic vertebrae, from GV-12 to GV-8, are considered very important as treatment points for nervous disorders. This refers to various psychosomatic and stress-related symptoms, including insomnia and irritability. Shiroda Bunshi's *Basic Study of Acupuncture and Moxibustion Therapy* also mentions nervous disorders as an indication for GV-11. Among the classics, *Gatherings from Outstanding Acupuncturists* by Gao Wu lists elation-despondency and forgetfulness-fright as indications for GV-11. In *Meridian Therapy for Acupuncture and Moxibustion,* Okabe Sodo suggests that patients with nervous disorders feel no pain when direct moxibustion is applied on intervertebral points between the third and eighth thoracic vertebrae, and that once they feel the heat, their condition improves. Okabe called these 'nerve points' *(shin kei ten/shén jīng diǎn)*. It is, in fact, true that reactions tend to appear at points of the Governing vessel in the upper back when patients have autonomic dysfunctions or psychosomatic disorders. This reaction appears most often at GV-10 or GV-11. Therefore, you can determine the level of stress a patient is under based upon the presence of a reaction at these points. If there is a marked reaction, the patient is worried about something or is under some stress.

There is a joke in Japan involving the opening line used by a fortune teller who says, "You have problems which you cannot tell anyone else, do you not?" It seems, however, that reaction at GV-11 tends to appear just when a patient has such problems. Rather than asking directly, "Have you been worried about something?," it is better to ask, "Have you been under some stress?"

The face of a patient who has been suffering from insomnia often resembles that of a fox, with the corners of the eyes raised. After treatment, including direct moxibustion on reactive Governing vessel points on the back, they will improve and the expression on their face will soften. Just one look, and it is obvious that they are better.

Thin people whose spines protrude tend not to have clear reactions at Governing vessel points. In such cases, reactions must be sought and treated on the lateral border of the spinous processes, or along the first line of the Bladder meridian. In my experience, however, it is more effective to treat nervous conditions by applying moxibustion on reactive points between the spinous processes (GV-9 to GV-11) than to treat the points on the side of the spinous processes or on the Bladder meridian.

GV-10 (*rei-dai / líng tái*)

LOCATION: Between the spinous processes of the sixth and seventh thoracic vertebrae (Fig. 2-25).

PALPATION: Locate with the patient in a prone position, using the same technique as described for GV-11.

INSERTION: Use the same technique as described for GV-11.

INDICATION: Nervous disorders, chest pain, coughing, wheezing.

GV-9 (*shi-yō / zhì yáng*)

(SYSTEMATIC): "In the joint under the seventh vertebra. Locate with the patient in a prone position."

(ILLUSTRATED): "On the back inferior to the spinous process of the seventh thoracic vertebra."

LOCATION: Between the spinous processes of the seventh and eighth thoracic vertebrae (Fig. 2-25).

PALPATION & INSERTION: Use the same technique as described for GV-11.

INDICATION: Nervous disorders and gastrointestinal diseases. Along with BL-17 just next to it, GV-9 is effective for the sensation of food being stuck or a blockage in the esophagus.

GV-6 (*seki-chū / jǐ zhōng*)

(*SYSTEMATIC*): "In the joint under the eleventh vertebra. Locate with the patient in a prone position."

LOCATION: Between the spinous processes of the eleventh and twelfth thoracic vertebrae (Fig. 2-26).

PALPATION: With the patient in a prone position, locate the spinous process of the fourth lumbar vertebra at the intersection of the Governing vessel and the line connecting the top of the iliac crests (which usually intersects the spinous process of

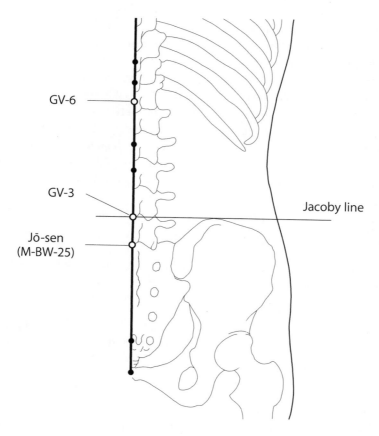

Fig. 2-26

69

the fourth lumbar vertebra). Then count superiorly to find GV-6 between the eleventh and twelfth thoracic vertebrae. GV-6 can also be located at the intersection of the Governing vessel and an imaginary line drawn between the acromion and the superior-lateral end of the iliac crest on the opposite side. A reaction that is found between the spinous processes of the lower thoracic vertebrae can be considered to be GV-6 and can be treated.

INDICATION: Apply direct moxibustion when the patient is a diabetic and there is a reaction at GV-6.

DISCUSSION: I started looking for reactions at GV-6 after I learned about the relationship between this point and diabetes in *Stories from a Moxibustion Practice* by Fukaya (1966). It is true that reactions often appear at GV-6 or one of the other lower thoracic interspinal points in diabetics. Therefore, when there is a strong reaction at one of these points, one can suspect that there is sugar in the urine. However, there are diabetics who do not show this reaction, so this diagnosis cannot be determined solely by palpating GV-6.

A certain elderly acupuncturist in my prefecture had been a diabetic for many years. One day I decided to see if he had a reaction at GV-6. He was wearing a suit, so I guessed at the location based on the intersection between the Governing vessel and a line from the acromion to the iliac crest on the opposite side. I found one place on the spine that was depressed. I poked my finger there and it seemed to sink right in. He exclaimed "That really hurts!" The reaction could be detected even with him fully clothed, so it was quite strong. His condition was also quite advanced.

GV-3 (*yō-kan / yáng guān*)

(*BASIC QUESTIONS*): "In the space beneath the sixteenth vertebra. Locate with the patient in a seated position."

(*ILLUSTRATED*): "On the lower margin of the spinous process of the fourth lumbar vertebra. The midpoint of the line connecting the iliac crests falls on the lower margin of the spinous process of the fourth lumbar vertebra, so it [GV-3] is in the depression just below."

LOCATION: In the depression below the intersection of the Governing vessel and the line connecting the top of the iliac crests (Fig. 2-26).

PALPATION: Strike lightly or press back and forth with the middle finger in the depression. The point is found where it is mushy or tender.

INSERTION: Use a vertical, shallow insertion. An intradermal needle or direct moxibustion can be applied instead.

INDICATION: Lower back pain and sciatica.

M-BW-25 (*jō-sen / shí qī zhuī xià*)

M-BW-25 is a miscellaneous point that was named Above the Sacrum (*jō-sen*) and made popular in Japan by Akabane. It is called Below the Seventeenth Vertebra (*shí qī zhuī xià*) in China.

(AKABANE, 1954): "On the posterior median line between the [spinous process of the] fifth lumbar vertebra and the sacrum."

LOCATION: On the Governing vessel between the fifth lumbar vertebra and the sacrum (Fig. 2-26).

PALPATION: The depression on the posterior median line just below the line connecting the top of the iliac crests is GV-3, and M-BW-25 is one more vertebra beneath GV-3. It is between the fifth lumbar vertebra and the sacrum, and this space tends to be a little larger than that between the lumbar vertebrae. Press the middle finger into this depression and move it back and forth or up and down. Percussion or lightly striking the point is another good way to find a reaction.

When patients with lower back pain are *not* tender at M-BW-25, probe to the side of the point. You will often find a reactive point just on the edge of the spinous process that makes the patient jump. To find this reactive point, use the middle finger to press in toward the spine from the side of the spinous process; press down this line on both sides onto the sacrum. Sometimes it is just next to the spinous process, and at other times, next to the intervertebral space.

INSERTION: Apply multiple cones of direct moxibustion for lower back pain with damage to an intervertebral disk or ligament. An intradermal needle may be retained instead. When the reaction is lateral to M-BW-25, a needle can be inserted vertically 0.5 to one unit to produce a good needle sensation.

INDICATION: Lower back pain with a herniated intervertebral disk, sciatica, urogenital diseases, hemorrhoids.

DISCUSSION: Whenever patients come in with lower back pain, I examine the midline above the sacrum and often find a depression, bulge, or tender point at either M-BW-25 or GV-3. The active point can be treated with acupuncture or moxibustion. One may find many active points on the back, however, and wish to limit the number of points to be treated. In this case, M-BW-25 or the adjacent point is preferred when the lower back pain is only in the center, there is extreme tenderness, and the patient has difficulty bending forward and backward.

When there is damage to an intervertebral disk or ligament, acupuncture alone does not help. Multiple cone moxibustion (over 15 cones) is required. Then the pain quickly subsides. When the back pain is still strong the day after treatment, close examination often reveals that the tender point in the intervertebral space that received moxibustion the day before is gone, or at least greatly reduced. Instead, the reaction often appears in the intervertebral space just above or below.

In the early days of my practice, a young man came in almost crawling with acute lower back pain which he got while digging up root vegetables. The area around M-BW-25 was visibly bulging. It was extremely painful when I pressed the point. There were no other reactive points (or I should say, at that time I was unable to find any). The pain disappeared completely after I applied 20 cones of moxa. Thirty-five years later, this patient still comes in from time to time with lower back pain. It is interesting that, even after all these years, M-BW-25 remains the most reactive point.

GV-2 (*yō-yu* / *yāo shū*)

(*SYSTEMATIC*): "Below the twenty-second vertebra."

(*ILLUSTRATED*): "Inferior to the fourth sacral segment. Sliding the finger superiorly from the tip of the coccyx with the patient in a prone position, about three units up you can feel the depression of the sacral hiatus. It is just medial and inferior to the fourth sacral foramina or BL-34."

(*WANG, 1165*): "In the deep depression. Locate this point on the back with the patient lying face-down and the body relaxed; both hands must be placed under the forehead, and the torso must be straight."

LOCATION: Between the sacrum and the coccyx (Fig. 2-27).

PALPATION: Slide the finger superiorly from the coccyx, and when the finger falls into the depression, press with a small circular motion to find a reaction.

INSERTION: Use a vertical, shallow insertion.

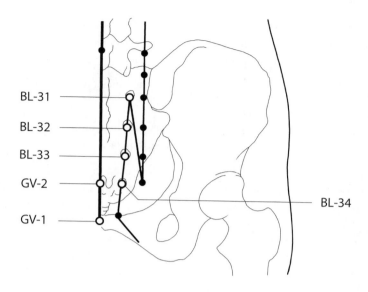

Fig. 2-27

INDICATION: Use acupuncture for hemorrhoids and coccygeal pain. Direct moxibustion is effective for constipation.

DISCUSSION: Patients sometime complain of pain in the coccyx unrelated to movement. When there is no reaction at GV-2 or GV-1 at the tip of the coccyx despite the presence of this type of pain, there is often a reaction at BL-32. Needling this point usually relieves the pain.

BL-12 (*fū-mon / fēng mén*)   ★★

(SYSTEMATIC): "On either side of the bottom of the second vertebra; each [is] located one-and-a-half units [from the midline]."

(ILLUSTRATED): "One-and-a-half units lateral to the point below the spinous process of the second thoracic vertebra."

(ACUPUNCTURE): "On the mid-interscapular line at the level of the space between the spinous processes of the second and third thoracic vertebrae. The mid-interscapular line is a vertical line that is midway between the medial border of the scapula and the median line."

LOCATION: 1.5 units lateral to the space between the spinous processes of the second and third thoracic vertebrae (Fig. 2-28).

PALPATION: Locate this point with the patient in a seated or prone position. Place the tip of the middle finger on the point and make small circles, or move it back and forth sideways.

INSERTION: Use a vertical, shallow insertion of 0.2 to 0.3 unit. When it is retained, the needle lays down on the skin. Contact needling is also beneficial.

INDICATION: Upper respiratory tract infection when there is sneezing, nasal discharge, or a sore throat. In the course of time, as the infection moves down toward the bronchi, the reaction also moves down the back points to BL-13 and BL-15, and finally to BL-17.

BL-12 is also effective for cervical spine conditions and spasms of the cervical muscles ('crick' in the neck) when movement of the neck is painful. In acute cases with fever or intense pain in the neck and upper back, retain needles superficially in BL-12 with the patient lying in a prone position. I once treated a patient with a crick in the neck by retaining needles in his upper back. The next day the pain was worse and he even had a slight fever. The needles must have been too deep. So, for the next treatment, I only did superficial needling, and did not retain any needles. The pain promptly subsided.

BL-13 (*hai-yu / fèi shū*)

(*SYSTEMATIC*): "On either side of the bottom of the third vertebra; each [is] located one-and-a-half units [from the midline]."

(*ILLUSTRATED*): "One-and-a-half units lateral to the point below the spinous process of the third thoracic vertebra. In most cases, the points on the first line of the Bladder meridian from BL-12 and BL-13 down to BL-23 in the lumbar area are located in the middle of the erector spinae muscles, and a thick muscle fiber can be palpated inside [the point]."

LOCATION: 1.5 units lateral to the space between the spinous processes of the third and fourth thoracic vertebrae (Fig. 2-28).

PALPATION: Locate this point with the patient in a seated or prone position, but it is easier to locate when the patient is seated. Find an induration by pressing with the

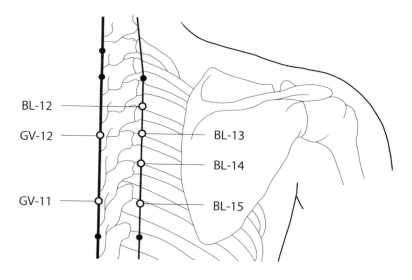

Fig. 2-28

tip of the middle finger and moving it back and forth sideways. In the interscapular area, indurations and tender points appear most often between BL-13 and BL-15, and next around BL-43. The quality of the reaction between BL-13 and BL-15, however, seems to be different from that around BL-43. For further explanation, refer to the discussion under BL-43.

INSERTION: Use a vertical, superficial insertion. The needle should reach the induration even though the insertion must be kept as shallow as possible. There will be a needle sensation that radiates superiorly to GB-21 and GB-20 when the needle tip reaches the induration. When there is an arthritic condition in the upper half of the body, over 10 cones of direct moxibustion will relieve the inflammation in the joint.

INDICATION: A reaction appears around BL-13, especially when there is inflammation in the upper half of the body. BL-13 is also effective for *katakori* (neck and shoulder stiffness), respiratory diseases, and intercostal neuralgia.

DISCUSSION: When there is pain and restriction in a joint of the upper half of the body, such as the shoulder joint, one might consider it to be a case of bursitis. Anyone can tell it is a case of frozen shoulder once movement in the shoulder becomes very limited. However, in the very early stages, it is often hard to tell if it is

75

a case of bursitis or arthritis, or a combination of the two. Even if medical tests show no rheumatoid reaction, it does not necessarily rule out rheumatoid arthritis. I often hear of cases where the joint swells up terribly after physical therapy or therapeutic exercise. If you are not sure whether it is bursitis or arthritis, check for a reaction around BL-13. If there is a substantial induration, most likely there is inflammation inside the joint. In addition, almost always, the point is tender. In cases of bursitis, there is rarely induration or tenderness around BL-13.

It was the moxibustion master Fukaya Isaburo who first pointed this out, and this is one of the hallmarks of Fukaya-style moxibustion, that is, a reaction appearing around BL-13 when there is arthritis anywhere in the upper half of the body, from the fingers and hand up to the jaw. The presence of induration and tenderness around BL-13 directly correlates to the degree of inflammation in the joints of the upper body. Thus, one can assess the extent of pathology as long as there is an obvious induration. Even if there are no symptoms, one can assume that the root of the disease is present. One can, therefore, prevent the outbreak of arthritis and the exacerbation of an existing condition by applying moxibustion.

The treatment of reactions around BL-13 from arthritis will be ineffective unless direct moxibustion is used. Acupuncture gives poor results, and even the average dose of five cones of moxa does not give quick results. Immediate results are achieved when the dose is doubled, that is, apply at least 10 cones or more (if possible) of direct moxibustion.

There was a time when it was common for unlicensed moxibustion practitioners, mostly old men practicing in their own homes, to apply huge cones of direct moxibustion. Almost invariably they used points on the back and lumbar area. One woman who came to me with joint pain in her shoulders and hands told me that she had gone to such a practitioner, and that her pain went away completely when he finished the moxibustion. I checked and there were six large moxa scars on her back associated points. Even though these practitioners were unlicensed, they got results, so people went to them. In Japan, there are secret family styles of moxibustion that are still practiced, and a similar shotgun approach is used. Considering the success of Fukaya-style moxibustion, however, one cannot dismiss direct moxibustion on the back-associated points by nonprofessionals as foolish folk remedies.

Interestingly enough, no induration can be found between BL-13 and BL-15 in cases of tennis elbow or trigger finger. Of course, it is useless to treat these points when there is no reaction. In Fukaya-style moxibustion, they look for reactions around BL-17 to treat arm pain from causes other than arthritis.

76

BL-14 *(ketsu-in-yu / jué yīn shū)*　　　★★★

(SYSTEMATIC): "On either side of the bottom of the fourth vertebra; each [is] located one-and-a-half units [from the midline]."

(ILLUSTRATED): "One-and-a-half units lateral to the point below the spinous process of the fourth thoracic vertebra."

LOCATION: 1.5 units lateral to the space between the spinous processes of the fourth and fifth thoracic vertebrae (Fig. 2-28).

PALPATION: When treating patients in the prone position, place a small pillow between their chin and CV-22, with their arms up around the pillow. Otherwise you can place the pillow under their chest so that they face straight down. It is convenient to locate points on the back in this position because points on both the upper and lower back can be treated at once. Another, simpler solution is to use a face cradle. When you want to be especially careful about locating BL-14, however, it is best to palpate with the patient seated. Use the same technique as described for palpating BL-13, that is, press with the middle finger and move it back and forth sideways.

INSERTION: Use a vertical, superficial insertion.

INDICATION: Same as those for BL-13 and BL-15. In other words, BL-14 is a point that connects to and can be substituted for BL-13 and BL-15.

BL-15 *(shin-yu / xīn shū)*　　　★★★

(SYSTEMATIC): "On either side of the bottom of the fifth vertebra; each [is] located one-and-a-half units [from the midline]."

(ILLUSTRATED): "One-and-a-half units lateral to the point below the spinous process of the fifth thoracic vertebra."

LOCATION: 1.5 units lateral to the space between the spinous processes of the fifth and sixth thoracic vertebrae (Fig. 2-28).

PALPATION: Same as that for BL-14. Use the middle finger and move it back and forth sideways.

INSERTION: Use a vertical or diagonal, shallow insertion. The best effects are obtained when BL-15 is needled shallowly, and a mild and pleasant needle sensation radiates to the top of the shoulder and to the pectoral region.

INDICATION: Heart disease, chest pain, palpitations, arrythmias, nervous disorders, and shortness of breath. The reaction in the above cases appears most often on the left side. The reaction can also appear on the right when there is coughing or other respiratory symptoms. Just as with BL-13, reactions can appear at BL-15 in cases of arthritis in the upper half of the body. The area between BL-13 and BL-15, and sometimes down to BL-16, can thus be regarded as one continuous field for this reaction. I usually treat only one set of active associated points in this whole field. Nevertheless, when the reaction is extensive, or long on the vertical axis, I locate the two most indurated points on the affected side and apply moxibustion to them.

DISCUSSION: There is a Japanese saying, "The grains of sand on a beach may be counted, but the causes of worry are endless." One need not mention the recent economic woes, as life in Japan has always been stressful with family, social, and business obligations. People with yin constitutions are sensitive, and they worry constantly. They react completely differently from those with yang constitutions, who are sometimes so happy-go-lucky that they don't worry even when they don't know where their next meal is coming from. When a person worries constantly, this is called 'laboring the heart' *(shin-ro)* in Japanese. The back becomes tense on the left side when there is a lot of mental stress. Palpation reveals a series of indurations and tender points on the left side from BL-13 down to BL-20. If these indurations and tender points are not relieved, the back begins to feel oppressively tight and this sensation spreads to the left pectoral region. Some patients become worried and go in for ECG tests just to be told that they are normal and there is nothing to worry about. Sometimes they receive the nebulous diagnosis of 'autonomic dysfunction'. They pretend that they are not worried because they want to believe they are fine, even though they do not feel fine. Other patients become infuriated because no one seems to understand what they are going through.

Even if it does not show up on the ECG, it is not good to allow such tension to become chronic. Eventually, abnormalities will appear on the ECG, and a person will have to carry nitroglycerin around. When the abnormal tension in the back is relieved with acupuncture and moxibustion, the oppressive sensation also disappears. When a needle is inserted in BL-15 and the tip reaches just the right point, there is a sensation in the area of the chest that had previously felt uncomfortable. This sensation is soothing and remarkably effective in alleviating the discomfort.

As long as the needle is inserted shallowly, there is no problem. It is dangerous, however, to insert a needle deeply in the back in an attempt to produce such a sensation in the chest. Deep insertion can cause pneumothorax, and the classics warn against this and other major complications:

> Inserting and penetrating the heart, death will ensue in one day. The reaction of belching will be caused. Inserting and penetrating the lungs, death will ensue in three days. The reaction of coughing will be caused. Inserting and penetrating the liver, death will ensue in five days. The reaction of talking [deliriously] will be caused. Inserting and penetrating the kidneys, death will ensue in six days. The reaction of sneezing will be caused. Inserting and penetrating the spleen, death will ensue in ten days. The reaction of heartburn will be caused. (*Basic Questions*, Chapter 52)

It is easy to imagine how such accidents might have occurred quite often during the Han Dynasty when thick and long needles were used for acupuncture. Even today, special care has to be taken when thick and long Chinese-style needles are being used.

Tension on the left side of the back is most effectively relieved by using a few other points in combination with BL-15, such as CV-17, ST-12, KI-23, and the Axillary point on the left side. A better strategy would be to treat imbalances in the meridians, that is, to determine the basic pattern and give a root treatment. For example, when SP-3 and PC-7 are tonified for Spleen deficiency, the results will increase dramatically.

As the back associated point of the Heart, BL-15 treats diseases of the Heart. The qi of the Heart appears at BL-15 on the yang aspect, and CV-14 on the yin aspect. It can be assumed that the back associated point and the front alarm point interact constantly. In *Acupuncture Point Diagnosis*, Gai Guo-Cai recommends BL-14 as the diagnostic and treatment point for Heart disease. In my experience, in cases of heart problems, reactions appear more often at BL-15, and to a lesser extent at the Axillary point on the left. You can find out if the patient has a heart condition by palpating BL-15 and the Axillary point on the left, as well as CV-17 and CV-14. It is a great system that designated BL-15 as the associated point and CV-14 as the alarm point of the Heart. Perhaps the ancients thought that the effect of balancing the meridians alone was insufficient for diseases of the organs. It might be that the organ system was independent of the meridian system at one time, and the associated and alarm points were the treatment points for the organs. It does seem that, in general, the associated and alarm points are close to their corresponding organs, and reactions do appear most readily at these points.

> The place that draws qi from the organs and [where the qi] pours [into] is known as the associated [points]. In general the abdomen is distant from the organs, and the back is close to the organs. Thus, the abdomen is needled and primarily moxibustion is applied on the back. In this way, the back has places where the qi of the organs collects. These are therefore called associated [points]. (Okamoto, 1693)

This passage implies that the front alarm points are farther from the organs, so there is less chance for accidentally puncturing an organ, and that the qi of the organs collects at the associated points. However, moxibustion is thought to be safer than acupuncture. No doubt this formulation is based on the passage above quoted from *Basic Questions*.

BL-17 (*kaku-yu* / *gé shū*)

(*SYSTEMATIC*): "On either side of the bottom of the seventh vertebra; each [is] located one-and-a-half units [from the midline]."

(*ILLUSTRATED*): "One-and-a-half units lateral to the point below the spinous process of the seventh thoracic vertebra. In many cases, thick muscle fibers can be palpated."

LOCATION: 1.5 units lateral to the space between the spinous processes of the seventh and eighth thoracic vertebrae (Fig. 2-29).

PALPATION: The spinous process of the seventh thoracic vertebra is on the line connecting the inferior angle of the scapulae, or just above or below it, so it is easy to find. Bear in mind that reactions at back associated points between BL-17 and BL-25 tend to appear slightly lateral compared to those above this region. In general, the associated points below BL-13 are located with the patient in a prone position, but if they are difficult to locate, ask the patient to sit up.

INSERTION: Use a superficial insertion with the needle pointed diagonally downward. When the right point is reached, a sensation sometimes radiates superiorly to the shoulders and above. As a rule, insert all needles in the back shallowly. It is best to get rid of the notion that deep insertion is necessary for a good response. When a patient is having an asthma attack in particular, pneumothorax is possible, even if you insert needles shallowly. I hear that some practitioners angle the needle medially to avoid this danger, but I still wonder if it is really necessary to insert deeply.

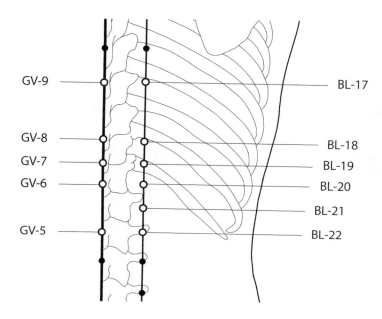

Fig. 2-29

INDICATION: This is the associated point of the diaphragm. Diseases of the diaphragm refer to difficulty in getting food down, as well as food getting stuck in the esophagus, and a tendency to vomit. Therefore, BL-17 is used for obstructions above the stomach whether the patient has an appetite or not. It is also the influential point for blood, and thus can be used for blood disorders. Reactions do tend to appear at BL-17 when women have dysmenorrhea or when they become perimenopausal. SP-6 and BL-17 should accordingly be checked on all women patients just to make sure.

BL-18 *(kan-yu / gān shū)*

(SYSTEMATIC): "On either side of the bottom of the ninth vertebra; each [is] located one-and-a-half units [from the midline]."

(ILLUSTRATED): "One-and-a-half units lateral to the point below the spinous process of the ninth thoracic vertebra. Locate in thick muscle fibers."

LOCATION: 1.5 units lateral to the space between the spinous processes of the eighth and ninth thoracic vertebrae (Fig. 2-29).

PALPATION: Use the same technique as discussed for BL-17. Palpate by moving the middle finger back and forth horizontally.

INSERTION: Use a diagonal, superficial insertion. The needle points downward, as with BL-17.

INDICATION: BL-18 is used when there is a Liver meridian imbalance and a reaction appears at this point. In cases with liver disease, the point is often reactive on the right side, and sometimes a protrusion or excess body hair is visible. When the chief complaint is pain or stiffness in the mid-back and there is a strong reaction at BL-18, liver disease can be suspected. BL-18 is also used for autonomic disorders like insomnia, and arthritic knee problems without edema.

BL-19 (tan-yu / dǎn shū)

(SYSTEMATIC): "On either side of the bottom of the tenth vertebra; each [is] located one-and-a-half units [from the midline]."

(ILLUSTRATED): "One-and-a-half units lateral to the point below the spinous process of the tenth thoracic vertebra."

LOCATION: 1.5 units lateral to the space between the spinous processes of the tenth and eleventh thoracic vertebrae (Fig. 2-29).

PALPATION: Use the same technique as discussed for BL-18.

INSERTION: Insert the needle angled 45° downward. The needle may also be angled medially. The depth should be shallow, but at times I go as deep as half the length of a 40mm needle.

INDICATION: BL-19 on the right is useful for gallbladder disease. Moxibustion is also effective.

DISCUSSION: When a patient complains of heartburn, nausea, and distention in the pit of the stomach, one can suspect gallbladder disease. The pattern is often either:

- Liver deficiency and Gallbladder excess, or

- Spleen deficiency and Liver-Gallbladder excess.

In such cases, the superficial level of the left middle position of the pulses is often hard. Furthermore, there is often a strong reaction when pressing a point just to the right of GV-7. (This is located between the spinous processes of the tenth and eleventh thoracic vertebrae. Find it by counting up six spaces between the spinous processes above the line connecting the top of the iliac crests.) It is uncanny how consistently this reaction appears in cases of gallbladder disease. The reaction can actually appear slightly above or below, and on on either side of, GV-7. This is one of the M-BW-35 points, also known as the *huá tuō jiá jí* points. To check for a reaction, poke the side of the spine with the tip of the middle finger in a medial direction. When I also find tenderness at GB-34 on the right, as well as sensitivity to pinching at ST-19 or ST-20 on the right, there is a stong possibility of a gallbladder problem. Inserting a needle in the M-BW-35 point sometimes produces a sensation in the gallbladder area. Moxibustion is also effective. When there is a strong reaction, the M-BW-35 point works just as well, if not better than, BL-19.

BL-20 (*hi-yu / pí shū*)

(SYSTEMATIC): "On either side of the bottom of the eleventh vertebra; each [is] located one-and-a-half units [from the midline]."

(ILLUSTRATED): "One-and-a-half units lateral to the point below the spinous process of the eleventh thoracic vertebra."

LOCATION: 1.5 units lateral to the space between the spinous processes of the eleventh and twelfth thoracic vertebrae (Fig. 2-29).

PALPATION: Move the tip of the middle finger back and forth over the erector spinae muscles to find the hardest point. Sometimes, however, the point is found in a hollow or depression.

INSERTION: Use a vertical or diagonal insertion, with the needle aimed downward. The depth varies from shallow (5mm) to deep (2cm), as a relatively deep insertion is safe in this location. When just the right depth is reached, distention in the abdomen is relieved and movement can be felt in the upper or lower abdomen.

INDICATION: Use when there is a reaction and there is an imbalance in the Spleen meridian. BL-20 is also useful for focal distention in the abdomen that comes with gastrointestinal disorders. BL-17 can also be used for focal distention, but BL-20 is the point of choice when there is pain in the abdomen and either too great an appetite or a lack of appetite. BL-20 is also useful for knee problems with swelling in the joint. This point is especially suited for direct moxibustion at home. The Spleen facilitates the discharge of fluids. Therefore, BL-20 is used for edema (in the face or limbs), sloshing sounds in the abdomen when it is pressed (often a sign of poor absorption), diarrhea, as well as heart and kidney diseases. BL-20 is thus a point with a wide range of applications.

DISCUSSION: As just stated, my approach is to look for a reaction at BL-20 whenever I find an imbalance in the Spleen meridian. How can this point be used if one is not sure whether there is an imbalance in the Spleen meridian?

Essentially, the function of the Spleen is the process of digestion. The Spleen and Stomach constantly work together to transform food and fluids into postnatal qi, and to send this to all the organs. Thus, when the function of the Spleen declines, the whole body is affected. A good appetite and digestion is a sign of a healthy Spleen. Patients who have good Spleen function respond well to acupuncture treatment. When a patient has Lung or Spleen deficiency, however, it just takes longer to get the same results. This cannot be helped because they just do not have the vitality to recover. Such patients are either thin or their skin is thin, lacking in luster, or tends to be wrinkled. Some have problems with sleep. Some people with Spleen imbalances become sleepy in the afternoon, and have a hard time staying awake when they have to listen to complicated or boring talks. Be sure to treat BL-20 and Spleen meridian points to alleviate such problems.

BL-21 (*i-yu* / *wèi shū*)

(SYSTEMATIC): "On either side of the bottom of the twelfth vertebra; each [is] located one-and-a-half units [from the midline]."

LOCATION: 1.5 units lateral to the space between the spinous processes of the twelfth thoracic and first lumbar vertebrae (Fig. 2-29).

PALPATION: Use the same technique as discussed for BL-20.

INSERTION: See BL-20.

INDICATION: When there is a strong reaction at BL-21, use it as a supplemental or alternative point for BL-20.

BL-22 *(san-shō-yu / sān jiāo shū)* ★★

(SYSTEMATIC): "On either side of the bottom of the thirteenth vertebra; each [is] located one-and-a-half units [from the midline]."

(ILLUSTRATED): "One-and-a-half units lateral to the point below the spinous process of the first lumbar vertebra. Applying strong pressure, there is a point in the muscle with a penetrating pain."

LOCATION: 1.5 units lateral to the space between the spinous processes of the first and second lumbar vertebrae (Figs. 2-29 and 2-30).

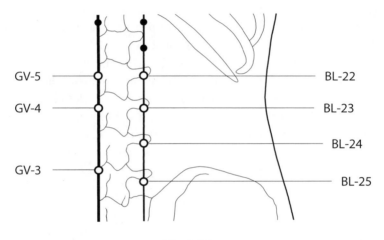

Fig. 2-30

PALPATION: Use the same technique as discussed for BL-20. Sometimes I find BL-22 by having the patient arch his back by propping himself up with his elbows. Flexion of the back muscles in this way makes the induration easier to find. I may also try light percussion on this point.

INSERTION: Use a vertical, shallow (5mm) to deep (2cm) insertion.

INDICATION: Used as a supplemental or alternative point to BL-23, BL-22 is effective for low-grade fevers from nephritis or pyelonephritis. BL-22 is also useful for poor elimination of fluids and spontaneous lower back pain. Retain an intradermal needle in BL-22 for school children with orthostatic albuminuria.[5]

DISCUSSION: The treatment of spontaneous lower back pain (pain without movement) is a little tricky. I usually treat patients in the side-lying position when there is a disk lesion or sciatica. I do not use many points. I like to press a point to see if it reduces or removes the pain. If it does, it is going to be a beneficial point, and so I retain a needle there to see how it affects the pain. Sometimes that is all it takes to relieve the pain, and at other times the pain gets worse. The reaction to needling the point varies considerably. There are times when many cones of direct moxibustion at just one point brings great relief. The key is to treat each point individually and with great care. When you use many points at once, the pain often gets worse and you get yourself into trouble.

Another kind of spontaneous lower back pain that occurs quite often is caused by stones in a kidney or ureter. In bad cases, the patient's face is drawn and the body becomes contorted; just watching this kind of patient is painful. The patient will jump with pain when you lightly strike BL-22 or BL-23 with your knuckles. Therefore, one must be sure to strike the points very gently. When light percussion like this causes pain, it is quite likely that kidney stones are moving down the ureter. The treatment point is either BL-22 or BL-23. Inserting a needle to a depth of about 40mm will result in a needle sensation that will reach the most painful place. This, however, is the direct method. There is an indirect method that is safer and more effective. Doing a root treatment is the best way. In other words, tonification points such as SP-3, LU-9, or KI-7 should be needled superficially first, before needling the back points.

BL-23 (*jin-yu / shèn shū*)

(*SYSTEMATIC*): "On either side of the bottom of the fourteenth vertebra; each [is] located one-and-a-half units [from the midline]."

(*ILLUSTRATED*): "One-and-a-half units lateral to the point below the spinous process of the second lumbar vertebra."

LOCATION: 1.5 units lateral to the space between the spinous processes of the second and third lumbar vertebrae (Fig. 2-30).

PALPATION: Points on the first line of the Bladder meridian from BL-23 and below tend to appear slightly medial to the points above. Use the tip of the middle finger to press toward the spine. Also check for pain with percussion.

INSERTION: Use a vertical, shallow (5mm) to deep (2cm) insertion.

INDICATION: Use BL-23 when there is an imbalance in the Kidney meridian. It is therefore good for symptoms such as dizziness, tinnitus, hearing loss, lack of energy, and tendency to tire easily. BL-23 is also useful for kidney diseases, hemorrhaging in internal organs, and poor elimination of fluids.

BL-25 *(dai-chō-yu / dà cháng shū)* ★★

(SYSTEMATIC): "On either side of the bottom of the sixteenth vertebra; each [is] located one-and-a-half units [from the midline]."

(ILLUSTRATED): "One-and-a-half units lateral to the point below the spinous process of the fourth lumbar vertebra."

LOCATION: 1.5 units lateral to the space between the spinous processes of the fourth and fifth lumbar vertebrae (Fig. 2-30).

PALPATION: Press with the middle finger and move the fingertip back and forth over the muscle. When there is a reaction, you will feel something hard, almost like cartilage or a piece of jerky. The point is worth using when there is one point that is indurated in this way. When the entire area is stiff and rigid like a board, as often happens in cases of lower back pain, it is difficult to differentiate any of the points. In that case, change the angle of the feet, bend the knees more, or have the patient lie on their side to somehow relax the back muscles. The hardest point must be located within the area that is tense. It is often difficult to find an induration unless you use strong pressure. One can press with the tip of the thumb to apply more pressure, but the thumb is not as sensitive, and this makes it hard to palpate the point. My technique is to double up my index finger behind my middle finger and press with a small circular or cross-fiber motion.

INSERTION: Use a vertical insertion. The needle can go in very deeply at this point, but I generally get good results at a depth of between 15 to 30mm. When I feel the needle tip hit the hard spot, patients often comment that they feel a sensation deep in their back or down their leg. If I continue to insert the needle beyond that point, suddenly the resistance I felt at the needle tip disappears and the sensation also goes away. The effect is lost along with the sensation.

INDICATION: Lower back pain, leg pain.

DISCUSSION: For herniated disks and back pain caused by pathology in the intervertebral joints, it is important to find and needle indurated points between BL-23 and BL-27. These indurations, however, are not always easy to locate. In my early years of practice, I had difficulty finding tender points and indurations around BL-25. I decided it was not an important point because I could not find a reaction. As I began to palpate more thoroughly, however, I found reactive points hiding deeper down. The reason it is difficult to find reactions here is because the entire low back area is tense in patients with lower back pain, and they tend to tighten up unconsciously as you palpate the affected area. Also, it is hard to feel active points when you press with the thumb. As I said in the description of BL-23, the tip of the middle finger is best suited for the work of pinpointing indurations. This is especially true for associated points on the lower end, like BL-26 and BL-27. Points in this area are essential for the treatment of lower back pain; it is therefore important to hone your palpation skills.

Iliac point *(chō-kotsu- ten / cháng gǔ diǎn)*   ★★★

LOCATION: This special point is located at the intersection of the iliac crest with a vertical line drawn on the medial border of the scapula. The intersection is near the lateral margin of the attachment of the erector spinae to the iliac crest (Fig. 2-31).

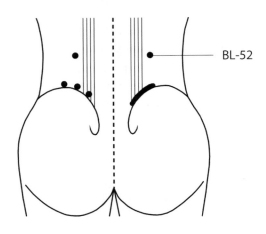

BL-52

Fig. 2-31

PALPATION: Find the lateral margin of the attachment of the erector spinae to the iliac crest. Probe the insertion of these muscles by pressing along the iliac crest in a medial direction with the middle finger. Press the tip of the finger into the muscle as if to dig in behind the iliac crest. Just pressing straight down does not work. Indurations can be located best by pressing just above the iliac crest with a downward slant of 30°. Move the fingertip back and forth in a cross-fiber motion. Indurations appear anywhere along the medial section of the iliac crest. Sometimes it is lateral to the intersection of the medial scapular line, but more often it is medial to the intersection. Indurations manifest as tight bands or lines of tension. The key is to work your fingertip back and forth as you press along the margin of the iliac crest.

INSERTION: Insert a 40mm, No. 0 or 1 needle diagonally and downward. When the sensation of qi is obtained, strong resistance can be felt at the tip of the needle at a depth of between 10 to 30mm. It feels like the muscle is grabbing the needle.

INDICATION: Myofacial back pain, especially back pain accompanying flexion or extension of the spine, chronic lower back pain, back pain in bedridden patients, sacroiliac disorders, inguinal pain, fatigue in the legs.

DISCUSSION: The Japanese representatives of the WHO Acupuncture Point Committee first reported on the new points and miscellaneous points submitted for inclusion in the WHO acupuncture point list of 1959. Among these was the miscellaneous point M-BW-23 (*yo gi/yāo yí*), which is very close to the point I have been using. Its location has been defined in the Japanese edition of *Acupuncture: A Comprehensive Text* as "three units lateral to the spinous process of the fourth lumbar vertebra" (Fig. 2-32). While the location is close to the point I use, it is not the same, so I decided to call my point the Iliac point. The Iliac point is not found in one specific location. It is usually medial to the medial scapular line, that is, second Bladder meridian line, but sometimes it corresponds to BL-25 or BL-26. Even though its location may vary, the defining characteristic of the Iliac point is that it is on the margin of the iliac crest.

The Iliac point is easy to locate on thin patients and hard to locate on obese ones. Sometimes you have to make an educated guess, but the effect is dramatic if you get the point just right. Quite often, the pain is resolved with just one needle. It is best to use a thin needle, such as a 40mm, No. 0 stainless steel needle or a No. 1 silver needle. Thin needles have to be inserted slowly and carefully. You cannot force your way in. You have reached the point when you feel some resistance or the needle becomes heavy. Even if the patient does not feel it at first, in a few moments

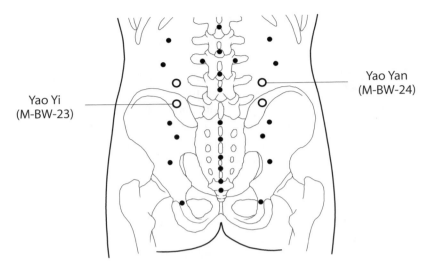

Fig. 2-32

they will feel a sensation reach the most painful area. This feeling of hitting the mark is wonderful, but hard to describe. The effect is nil if the needle passes right through the point without resistance.

A needle sensation is important for quick results, at least when in comes to the Iliac point. When the patient is muscular and there is no gap between the muscles and the iliac crest, you can use a slightly thicker needle, such as a 40mm, No.1 stainless steel needle. When the muscles along the iliac crest are uniformly tight, however, the Iliac point is usually not indicated. It is better to seek other points that show a clear difference by palpation.

The depth of insertion at the Iliac point varies and it has little to do with the build of the patient. Sometimes I've had to insert a needle as much as 60mm to reach the Iliac point. If you do not feel any resistance at the needle tip or the 'arrival of qi', withdraw the needle, palpate, and insert the needle again. Try needling the point up to three times, but no more. Otherwise, the pain could get worse the day after the treatment. Direct techniques can be very effective, but they can also have the opposite effect. There is much less danger with indirect techniques. A person who can quickly and precisely locate and needle the Iliac point may be considered a full-fledged practitioner. After a few treatments, the reaction at the Iliac point moves medially. Then it corresponds to points like BL-25 or BL-26.

Ever since I introduced the Iliac point in the *Journal of Japanese Acupuncture and Moxibustion* (Shudo, 1975), I have kept an eye out for references to similar points. The point that comes closest is 'lower back pain' *(yaō tòng)* noted in *Atlas of Off-Meridian Miscellaneous Points for Acupuncture* (Hao, 1973) (Fig. 2-33). Its location is described as being "two units lateral to the point between the spinous processes of the fourth and fifth lumbar vertebrae; half a unit lateral to BL-25." However, both this point and M-BW-23 mentioned above are described as specific points, and this differs from my concept of a line along the border of the iliac crest.

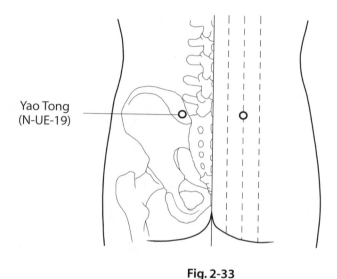

Yao Tong
(N-UE-19)

Fig. 2-33

BL-27 *(shō-chō-yu / xiǎo cháng shū)*　　　　★

(SYSTEMATIC): "On either side of the bottom of the eighteenth vertebra; each [is] located one-and-a-half units [from the midline]."

LOCATION: M-BW25 *(jōsen/shí qī zhuī xià)* is located between the fifth lumbar vertebra and the sacrum, and BL-27 is located 1.5 units lateral to this point, below the first sacral segment (Fig. 2-34).

PALPATION: The line connecting the tops of the iliac crest intersects the spine on or below the spinous process of the fourth lumbar vertebra. This line can be used to locate BL-25, BL-26, and BL-27 in succession. Otherwise, you can locate BL-27

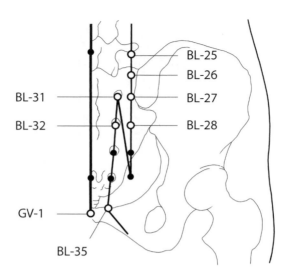

Fig. 2-34

by first locating BL-32 at the medial inferior corner of the posterior superior iliac spine, and then locating BL-31 just above it. BL-27 is located just lateral to BL-31. The reaction appears more medially as you go lower on the Bladder meridian.

INSERTION: Use the same technique as described for BL-25, except that it is not quite as deep.

INDICATION: Gynecological disorders, arthritis in lower limbs, hemorrhoids.

DISCUSSION: BL-26 lies between BL-25 and BL-27, and it seems to encompass the effect of both points. Thus, its indications include lower back pain and sciatica, as well as those noted above. Use BL-26 whenever it has a stronger reaction than the adjacent points.

BL-32 *(ji-ryō / cì liáo)*

(SYSTEMATIC): "[In] the second space. In the depression on either side of the spine [of the sacrum]."

LOCATION: In the second sacral foramina (Fig. 2-34).

PALPATION: There is a depression at the medial inferior corner of the posterior superior iliac spine that often feels soggy when pressed. Press vertically (downward toward the table) with the middle finger, adding a small circular motion.

INSERTION: Use a vertical insertion. It is best if the needle tip goes into the sacral foramen. If you have trouble getting the needle in, go over on the other side of the patient and angle the needle superiorly.

INDICATION: Urogenital diseases, hemorrhoids, coccygeal pain.

DISCUSSION: In his book *Stories from a Moxibustion Practice*, Fukaya Isaburo has the following to say about BL-32: "This is a tender point for sciatica and an indispensable point for stopping pain. If it is not effective, add BL-37."

BL-32 is also listed as a key point for neuralgia (sciatica) in Shiroda's *Basic Study of Acupuncture and Moxibustion Therapy*. On the other hand, Kinoshita Haruto states in *Treatment of Sciatica* that needling BL-32 exacerbates some cases of sciatica. Personally, I do not use BL-32 for sciatica, and so I cannot comment on this. However, it seems like there has to be other factors that come into play if practitioners are getting opposite results.

What comes immediately to mind when I mention BL-32 is hemorrhoids. Just a day after my peritonitis had cleared up when I was a teenager, my favorite baseball team came to play at a local ballpark. I just could not pass up the opportunity. I watched the game on the concrete steps of the outfield seats. Two or three days later, my anus felt funny, and I developed bleeding hemorrhoids that refused to heal. Finally, I received a diagnosis of anal fistula. I had the bandage replaced every day at a local hospital, but the lead pencil-sized opening would not close up. My doctor wanted to operate, but my acupuncturist Master Miura advised against it, because he said it would cause a relapse of my tuberculosis.

Soon after that, Master Miura gave me a thorough examination. I still recall the excruciating pain when he pressed around BL-32. It seemed like the whole area was one big tender point, and I clearly remember that pain to this day. Even after his treatment, rather than healing, five openings appeared around the anal fistula and I had a relapse of tuberculosis.

With the many openings in the fistula, it became impractical to go to the hospital to change the bandage all the time, so I used a mirror to change the bandage myself. Master Miura also gave me acupuncture. I do not remember the exact points, but he said it was in a depression next to BL-32. It may actually have been closer to BL-53. He used a 60mm needle, and inserted almost the entire length of the needle, which I could feel as a sensation in my anus. It was a sensation hard to describe, but it felt good. After repeated local treatments, I finally healed to a point where I no longer needed a bandage. The power of natural healing is remarkable.

BL-35 (*e-yō / huì yáng*) ★

(SYSTEMATIC): "On either side of the coccyx."

(ILLUSTRATED): "Half a unit to either side of the tip of the coccyx."

LOCATION: 0.5 unit lateral and slightly superior to the tip of the coccyx (Fig. 2-34).

PALPATION: With the patient in a side-lying position, ask them to extend their leg on the bottom and flex the leg on top (Fig. 2-35). Place the bent knee on the table and position yourself on the front side of the patient. Trace the border of the coccyx superiorly from the tip. Your finger will come to a stop midway. Press and move the fingertip back and forth to pinpoint the induration. The thinner the patient, the higher up the point will be.

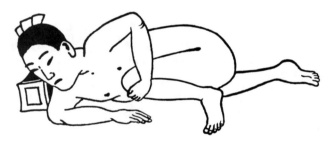

Fig. 2-35

INSERTION: Needle this point with the patient and practitioner positioned in the same way as noted above. A sensation will be felt in the anus once a depth of 50 to 60mm is reached. If the patient is thin, the sensation is felt at a depth of around 50mm. If there is a sensation somewhere other than the anus, withdraw the needle, palpate the point once more, and reinsert the needle. The needle must be thick; use one between No. 3 and No. 5.

INDICATION: Hemorrhoids. Needling the left side brings relief when defecation needs to be induced in cases of rectal disorders.

94

Gluteal point (*den-atsu*)

(*KINOSHITA, 1968*): "I will call the midpoint of a line drawn between the superior medial corner of the greater trochanter and the posterior superior iliac spine the Gluteal point *(denatsu)*."

LOCATION: At the midpoint between the greater trochanter and the posterior superior iliac spine (Fig. 2-36).

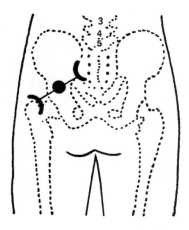

Fig. 2-36

PALPATION: This point can be located with the patient in a prone position. However, for the greatest accuracy, it is best to palpate it with the patient in a side-lying position. Find the point midway between the greater trochanter and the iliac spine in the middle of the gluteals. Firmly pressing the small mound with the tip of the middle finger or thumb, you can feel a hard spot. If you cannot feel anything, pinch the area to find a point that is slightly swollen, or where the skin is thicker. The patient will be more sensitive there. Abnormal hardness in the muscle (indurations) can be detected when you press deeply with the tip of the middle finger, or lightly strike the point with your knuckle.

INSERTION: Use a 50mm needle when needling the patient in the prone position. A 40mm needle is adequate when the patient is lying on the side. Insert the needle vertically right up to the induration. When the patient is lying on the side, the point comes closer to the surface and can be reached with a shallower insertion.

INDICATION: Sciatica, hemorrhoids, pathology of the piriformis muscle.

DISCUSSION: Even though their complaint is lower back pain, I find many patients are very sensitive when I pinch their Gluteal points. When this is the case, it can be assumed that the sciatic nerve is affected.

Sometimes patients complain of knee pain that bothers them at night. When I examine them and there is very little tenderness or signs of inflammation around the knee, but there is tenderness at the Gluteal point or BL-59, I assume they are feeling the sciatic pain in their knee. In cases like this, palpation of the Gluteal point serves a diagnostic purpose.

Once, my hemorrhoids returned and continued to bleed for a long time. Even slight anal bleeding is disturbing when it continues over a long period. When I attended a meeting of our local acupuncture association, I managed to talk a respected colleague, Kagiono Masashi, into giving me a treatment. He started by applying direct moxibustion on my low back and hip, and we discovered that the Gluteal point on the left hip did not feel any heat. He therefore burned a few dozen cones at this point until I could feel the heat. The next morning I found the bleeding had stopped. After two weeks of applying direct moxa at my Gluteal point, the heat sensitivity returned to normal.

BL-42 (haku-ko / pò hù)

(*BASIC QUESTIONS*): "Locate [it] with the patient seated with legs folded under."

(*WANG, 1027*): "In the deep depression."

(*SYSTEMATIC*): "On either side of the bottom of the third vertebra; each [is] located three units [from the midline]."

(*ILLUSTRATED*): "The points from BL-41 down to BL-54 are on the lateral margin of the erector spinae muscles, and they are four finger-widths lateral to the Governing vessel. The six points from BL-41 to BL-46 are often covered by the medial aspect of the scapula and [the patient must be positioned so that] the scapulae are spread apart. Bringing the elbows together as shown in *Difficult to Learn Point Locations* [Ishizaka, 1835] makes locating it easier." (Fig. 2-38)

LOCATION: Lateral to BL-13, on the medial border of the scapula when the arms are at the sides (Fig. 2-37).

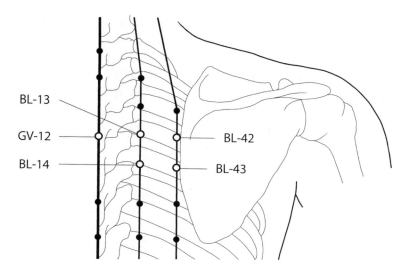

Fig. 2-37

PALPATION: Points on the back are usually located and treated with the patient lying in a prone position, but BL-41 and BL-42 are best located with the patient seated. Reactions tend to appear at these points when the patient crosses their arms.

INSERTION: Use a vertical or diagonal, shallow insertion, with the needle pointed superiorly. A needle sensation can be obtained with very shallow needling.

INDICATION: Numbness in arm, stiffness in neck, or inability to turn one's head due to pain.

DISCUSSION: The third Bladder meridian line begins with BL-41 and BL-42. The second Bladder meridian line begins with BL-12 and BL-13. The first Bladder meridian line is just next to the spinous processes, and points on this line are known as M-BW-35 or *huá tuō jiá jí* points. The points on the third line are considered to be supplemental to the back associated points on the second line. In other words, BL-41 is the supplemental point of BL-12, and is used in cases of the common cold and colds that are protracted. BL-42 is the supplemental point of BL-13, and is used for protracted respiratory ailments.

Points on the upper back are best located and needled with the patient in a prone position, but it takes some ingenuity to locate BL-42 when the patient is prone. Usually I have my patients place their hands on their head so their elbows come out to the side and their chest is flat against the table. This way the scapulae are spread apart. Nevertheless, the position in which these points show up most clearly is the seated position. It is even better if the patient brings the elbows together, because this makes indurations at BL-42 easy to find. The following explanation is given in *Difficult to Learn Point Locations*:

> When locating points for moxibustion, every time [have the patient] sit straight with legs folded under, and with the hands under the chin to support it [Fig. 2-38]. Be careful that [the patient] does not fall over. (Ishizuka, 1835)

Another method that I use is to have the patient cross the arms and reach to hold the opposite shoulders. This opens the space between the scapulae considerably (Fig. 2-39).

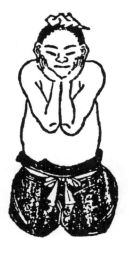 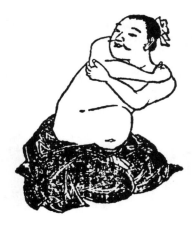

Fig. 2-38 **Fig. 2-39**

Shiroda (1940) and Irie (1980) listed BL-42 as a special point for visual disturbances when bright lights or "stars" are seen. This reminds me of my youngest sister who suffered from *katakori* (neck and shoulder stiffness) and eye problems, probably because she was a knitting teacher. Her eyes would become congested and painful, and she also had headaches and saw stars. These days they have medicated eye drops that work wonderfully, but rinsing and steaming the eyes were the only methods available fifty years ago, right after the war. However, my sister loved acupuncture and let me practice on her. I must have located and needled practically all of the 365 points on her. Every point I needled she said felt wonderful. I especially remember the indurations she had around BL-41 and BL-42. When I needled these points, she felt a sensation going up the back of her neck. The points that seemed to work especially well for my sister's *katakori* were BL-42, GB-21, and Upper BL-10.

BL-43 (*kō-kō-yu / gāo huāng shū*)

(SYSTEMATIC): "On either side of the bottom of the fourth vertebra; each [is] located three units [from the midline]."

LOCATION: Lateral to BL-14 on the medial edge of the scapula (Fig. 2-37).

PALPATION: Position the patient so the scapulae are spread apart.

- *Prone position.* Place a pillow under the patients' chin and have them hug it with both arms. It is best when the chest rests flat against the bed. The trapezius runs diagonally downward to attach to the medial border of the scapula, and so follow the muscle fibers and probe diagonally and superiorly with the tip of the middle finger. Also probe along the edge of the scapula, pressing superiorly and with a small circular motion. You will find an induration or tense strand of muscle tissue.

- *Seated position.* Have the patient cross their arms and press along the edge of the scapula, moving your fingertip back and forth horizontally.

INSERTION: Use a diagonal insertion with the needle pointed superiorly. I have a habit of giving my treatments from the left side of the table, so the needle tip points laterally as well as superiorly. This seems to work better. I try to keep the needle shallow, but sometimes when the needle tip reaches the induration, I find it has gone in half an inch.

INDICATION: Stiffness in the shoulders and back from overuse of the arms and hands. (The reaction tends to appear on the side of the dominant arm, and the amount of overuse can be estimated by the size and hardness of the induration.) BL-43 is also useful for fatigue and low-grade fevers from a cold.

DISCUSSION: This point is acclaimed by Suganuma in his book *Rules of Acu-*

puncture (1766): "Depletion and exhaustion, there is nothing among the one-hundred illnesses that cannot be cured. Truly this point is a godsend to doctors for urgent cases."

From my reading of the classics, it seems that BL-43 was widely used for extreme fatigue and malnourishment. This point still has wide application in the modern age. Needling BL-43 produces a sensation at GB-21 that extends superiorly toward GB-20, and sometimes even to the top of the head. As you needle the point, you can feel its marvelous effects, and it can make you salivate. Sometimes there is a fasciculation in the trapezius, and for a while the shoulder tension disappears.

BL-43 is ideal for so-called 'techno-stress' or computer work that involves eye strain and overuse of the hands. The location of BL-43 requires that one be careful about pneumothorax. Special caution is advised when needling BL-43 on patients during an asthma attack.

BL-50 (*i-sō / wèi cāng*)

(*SYSTEMATIC*): "On either side of the bottom of the twelfth vertebra; each [is] located three units [from the midline] in the depression."

LOCATION: 1.5 units lateral to BL-21 and three units lateral to the point between the spinous processes of the twelfth thoracic and first lumbar vertebrae (Fig. 2-40).

PALPATION: Find a tender point in the depression lateral to BL-21 just under the ribs.

INSERTION: Insert the needle about one unit (30mm) vertically or diagonally downward. If the patient is obese, you may need to use a 50mm needle and go a little deeper.

INDICATION: Stomach or abdominal pain.

BL-52 (*shi-shitsu / zhì shì*)

(*SYSTEMATIC*): "On either side of the bottom of the fourteenth vertebra; each [is] located three units [from the midline]. Locate with the patient sitting on folded legs."

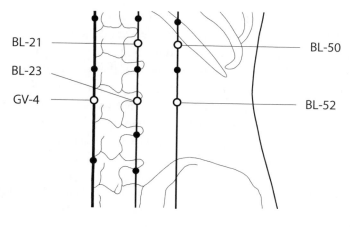

Fig. 2-40

LOCATION: The point is located three units lateral to GV-4, which is between the spinous processes of the second and third lumbar vertebrae, and 1.5 units lateral to BL-23 (Fig. 2-40).

PALPATION: A hard area can be detected by probing the back midway between the twelfth rib and the iliac crest using four fingers. Use a slight up-and-down (vertical) motion as you press. Press in small circles with the tip of the middle finger to find the hardest point. This point will be especially tender on thin patients. Be careful not to press too hard.

INSERTION: Use a diagonal insertion with the tip pointed in a medial and inferior direction. Use a 50mm needle and insert about one unit (30mm).

INDICATION: Fatigue, lower back pain, and kidney stones, as well as a supplemental point to BL-23 for urogenital diseases.

DISCUSSION: BL-52 is a point where, more often than not, there is tenderness or an induration. Sometimes the induration is anatomical and cannot be removed. However, when this induration is related to some pathology, it will also be tender and the hardness will feel different.

Soon after I began studying acupuncture, an old woman came to my teacher's place to get treatment while he was away. This was one of the first opportunities I had to treat someone unsupervised. Her main complaint was that of feeling bloated in the morning. Since I found indurations at BL-52, I applied multiple cones of direct moxibustion and needled BL-23, KI-6, and points above and below the navel. When the patient returned for another treatment, she told my teacher that my treatment worked very well, and I guess he had reason to be proud of me. I suppose I was saved by the indurations at BL-52 and how easy they are to palpate.

Sometimes, when patients with lower back pain have discomfort in the area around BL-52, the indurations can be difficult to palpate because the whole area is tight or the patient is obese. You can guess at the point and needle it, but it still may feel like you are not right on the point. Treat such patients on their side, and you will find it easier to locate and needle the induration. Under these circumstances, the point can be treated with a shorter 40mm needle. My patients report a pleasant sensation when I use a silver, 40mm, No. 1 or 2 needle. Sometimes, when the patient has discomfort around BL-52, reactions are found at BL-22 or BL-23 instead. Needling these points to a depth of about one unit often produces a strong sensation at BL-52.

BL-52 is one of the standard points of both the Sawada and the Ohta styles of acupuncture. The purpose of needling this point is to reinforce Kidney essence. The father of Ohta Rinsai, the leader of Ohta style acupuncture, is said to have needled this point every day on himself in the side-lying position.

BL-53 *(hō-kō / bāo huāng)*   ★

(SYSTEMATIC): "On either side of the bottom of the nineteenth vertebra; each [is] located three units [from the midline] in the depression. Locate with the patient prone."

(ILLUSTRATED): "Three units lateral to the point below the second sacral segment. With the patient in the prone position, locate BL-28, which is seven-tenths of a unit lateral to BL-32. BL-53 is one-and-a-half units lateral to BL-28, and all three points are in line. The flesh in this area is deep."

LOCATION: Lateral to BL-32 and BL-28, three units lateral to the median line (Fig. 2-41).

PALPATION: First locate BL-32 on the medial inferior corner of the posterior superior iliac spine. Palpate lateral to BL-32 on the border of the sacrum using three fingers. Move up and down across the insertion of the gluteal muscles to find an induration or depression.

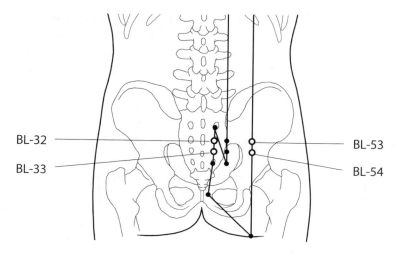

Fig. 2-41

INSERTION: Use a vertical or slightly diagonal insertion with a medial slant. I insert to a depth of three or four units for patients with prostate problems or loss of libido. This causes a deep, radiating sensation to the perineum, anus, inguinal area, or down to the feet.

INDICATION: Oliguria, loss of libido, prostate disease.

DISCUSSION: Years ago I co-authored an article with my colleague Nakamura Yaeko entitled "One-Needle Technique for Rejuvenation" (Nakamura, 1976). This was the first of my articles to be featured in the *Journal of Japanese Acupuncture and Moxibustion*. It was about deep insertion in the Rejuvenation point *(wakagaeri-ipponshin),* a point very close to BL-53. According to Nakamura, the Rejuvenation point is "in a depression four finger-widths lateral to the point [on the median line], three finger-widths above the tip of the coccyx." So for this use, the Rejuvenation point can be considered as an alternate location for BL-53.

To locate this point, instead of an induration, I look for a depression. The depth of insertion is up to four units, which is very deep. When patients see the needle, they are taken by surprise. It is no wonder, because my needling is generally quite shallow. Therefore, I keep the long needle out of their sight. I insert the needle into the depression close to BL-53, but I do not always hit the mark. Sometimes the needle runs up against bone and I have to reinsert it a few times before I get it right.

103

There is a radiating sensation when the needle is successfully inserted. Sometimes a sensation travels down the leg. This means the sciatic nerve has been stimulated, but this is not the aim of this technique. Correctly done, this deep insertion technique produces a sensation in the lower abdomen or in the penis for men.

Needling the Rejuvenation point has an amazing effect in improving libido. One patient told me that he had an erection all the way home. This effect does not last very long, but it is nonetheless quick and dramatic. Needling BL-53 this way is also effective for oliguria. One of my patients had an enlarged prostate and was having difficulty urinating. After I did the deep insertion technique, he was immediately able to urinate normally again. For a long time he continued to come for treatment once or twice a year, whenever he had difficulty urinating. He lived to a ripe age of over 80 without a prostate operation. Deep insertion at BL-53 is one technique you should try if a patient has oliguria.

BL-54 (*chip-pen / zhì biān*) ★

(SYSTEMATIC): "On either side of the bottom of the twenty-first vertebra; each [is] located three units [from the midline] in the depression. Locate with the patient prone."

(ILLUSTRATED): "Three units lateral to the point below the third sacral segment."

LOCATION: Lateral to BL-33 and three units from the median line (Fig. 2-41).

PALPATION: Palpate the muscles lateral to the sacrum at the level of BL-33. Press with three fingers and move them up and down across the muscles to find an induration.

INSERTION: Use a vertical, shallow (5mm) to deep (3cm) insertion.

INDICATION: Oliguria, hemorrhoids.

POINTS ON THE CHEST
AND ABDOMEN

CV-17 (dan-chū / dàn zhōng)

(SYSTEMATIC): "One-and-six-tenths unit inferior to CV-18, in the depression. Locate with the patient supine."

(ILLUSTRATED): "Between the nipples. It is a slightly depressed point at the mid-point of the line connecting the nipples. It is tender when pressed."

LOCATION: On the sternum in the center between the fourth intercostal spaces (Fig. 2-42).

PALPATION: Make a rough guess at the point between the nipples and press just above it with the tip of the middle finger. Work your way down the sternum in small increments to locate a depression or a soggy point. To palpate the point more precisely, make small circles with the fingertip to find the most tender point.

INSERTION: Use a diagonal, shallow insertion with the needle pointed downward.

INDICATION: Neurosis and psychosomatic conditions, heart disease, gastrointestinal disease, breast disease, insufficient lactation.

DISCUSSION: It seems that tenderness at CV-17 increases when people are depressed or feel pessimistic. When direct moxibustion is applied at CV-17, the tenderness diminishes, the chest feels more open, and the dark mood lifts. I used to apply moxibustion at CV-17, but since CV-17 is more sensitive and harder to treat, I stopped using it in favor of points with the same effect on the Governing vessel (GV-9 or GV-10). Now I use CV-17 primarily for diagnosis; tenderness at CV-17 and at the Axillary point on the left side is an important indicator of heart disease. However, I still apply direct moxibustion at CV-17 and SI-11 for insufficient lactation and mastitis. This works to soften the maxillary glands and facilitate lactation.

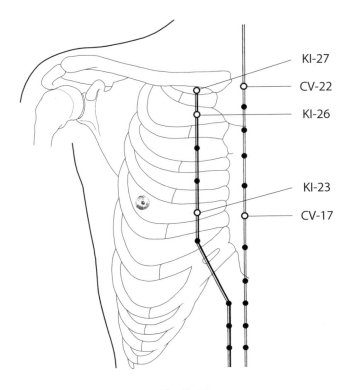

Fig. 2-42

When patients have gastrointestinal problems, they sometimes complain of a 'stuck' feeling in their throat or under their sternum. Needling CV-17 relieves this obstruction. I needle CV-17 together with CV-21 to relieve any discomfort in the esophagus. These points are very effective for cases of esophageal spasm, where food literally becomes stuck in the esophagus. CV-17 is the front alarm point of the Pericardium meridian, and treating the Pericardium meridian is effective for digestive problems as well as for circulatory problems.

KI-27 (*yu-fu / shū fŭ*)

(*SYSTEMATIC*): "Under the clavicle. Two units on either side of CV-22, in the depression. Locate with the patient supine."

106

(*ILLUSTRATED*): "On the inferior margin of the clavicle and two units from the median line, where the first rib begins to go under the clavicle and there is a depression."

LOCATION: Under the clavicle and close to the manubrium of the sternum (Fig. 2-42).

PALPATION: Place two fingers on the inferior margin of the clavicle and slide them medially toward the sternum. Pressing down, you can feel the point where the first rib rises up, and right next to it, you will find a tight strand of muscle that is tender.

INSERTION: Retain the needle superficially. The needle does not need to be inserted any further after tapping insertion with a tube.

INDICATION: Thoracic outlet syndrome (especially with hyperabduction syndrome),[6] throat and thyroid disorders.

KI-26 (*waku-chū / yù zhōng*)

(*SYSTEMATIC*): "One-and-six-tenths unit below KI-27, in the depression. Locate with the patient supine."

(*ILLUSTRATED*): "In the first intercostal space, two units lateral to the median line."

LOCATION: In the first intercostal space on the lateral margin of the sternum (Fig. 2-42).

PALPATION: The first rib is half hidden under the clavicle, so there is no groove between it and the clavicle. The groove or space between the ribs begins between the first and second rib, which is known as the first intercostal space. In the same manner as KI-27, place two fingers between the ribs. Find the point where the first rib joins the sternum and press and move the fingertips horizontally to find a tender point.

INSERTION: Use a vertical, shallow insertion.

INDICATION: Thoracic outlet syndrome, throat and thyroid disorders.

KI-23 (*shim-pō / shén fēng*)

(*SYSTEMATIC*): "One-and-six-tenths unit below KI-24, in the depression. Locate with the patient supine."

(ILLUSTRATED): "In the fourth intercostal space, two units lateral to the median line."

LOCATION: Lateral to CV-17 in the fourth intercostal space, on the margin of the sternum (Fig. 2-42).

PALPATION: At the intersection of the median line and the line connecting the nipples is CV-17. Place the ring finger in the fourth intercostal space, the index finger on the fifth rib just below, and the middle finger against the margin of the sternum. Press and move the middle finger up and down on the margin of the sternum to locate the most tender point.

INSERTION: Use a vertical, shallow insertion. Also, the needle may be inserted horizontally with the tip pointed laterally.

INDICATION: Costal neuralgia and on the left for heart disease.

Axillary point *(eki-ka-ten)*

(AKABANE, 1954): "Mark the point at the intersection of a vertical line from the center of the axilla and a horizontal line going through the nipples to the side. The point is about 8mm below the axilla. In addition, place two more marks, one above and one below, 2.5cm from the point. These shall be called the Axillary points."

LOCATION: Anterior to the intersection of the vertical axillary line and the mid-sternal line (horizontal line at the level of the nipples) (Fig. 2-43).

PALPATION: To locate the Axillary point on the right, place your middle finger on the approximate location of the Axillary point and move it toward the breast as you circle or move the fingertip back and forth. It is unusual for the reaction to appear on the axillary line; almost always, it is more anterior toward the breast. I find it appears most often around the midpoint between the axillary line and the nipple in the intercostal space. Check the points just above and below in the same manner. Use this same technique to locate the Axillary point on the left. You can try moving the fingertip up and down as you press. You can also place both middle fingers on the Axillary points on both sides at once. It is relatively easy to locate the best point when pressing on both sides this way, because the reactions can be compared.

INSERTION: Place an intradermal needle pointing posteriorly and perpendicular to the axillary line.

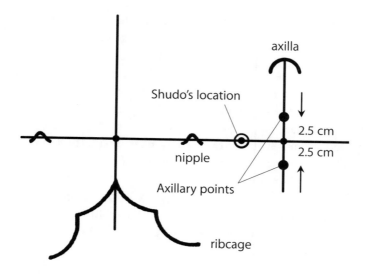

Fig. 2-43

INDICATION: Respiratory conditions including coughing, asthma, and breathing difficulties. I also often use it as a diagnostic and treatment point for heart disease.

DISCUSSION: I never used points around the axilla until the Axillary point was identified by Akabane. Once I began using it, I found it was very useful both for diagnosis and treatment. Usually, the reaction appears anterior to the axillary line. As is true with standard points, locating and treating the point with the greatest reaction is the most effective approach. When there is no reaction in the intercostal space, the point is sometimes hiding under the lower margin of a rib. So place the finger along the bottom edge of a rib and probe for the point by moving the fingertip back and forth horizontally.

Looking at an acupuncture point chart, you will find that SP-21 is on the axillary line, and closer to the breast is SP-18. The Axillary point does resemble the Spleen meridian points in some respects. The main indication given for these Spleen meridian points in the classics is pain in the flank region. There are some texts that mention asthma, but it is clear that Akabane's use of intradermal needles in the Axillary point made this application popular.

The Axillary point is effective for coughing, especially dry coughs with no phlegm. Even when there is phlegm, it will become thin and eventually disappear if you keep treating the Axillary point. In Akabane's approach, one is not supposed to

109

use the Axillary points on both sides at once. Only the side with the stronger reaction is used. Nevertheless, I tried treating both sides at the same time and found that it worked even better. Thus, when the coughing or asthma is severe, I use both sides, and when it starts to improve, I compare the reaction on both sides and place an intradermal needle only on the more sensitive side.

When pinching the skin around the Axillary point, the place where subcutaneous fat is the thickest seems to be the most sensitive. So, instead of pressing to find the reaction, one can pinch to locate the Axillary point. This technique is especially useful when a patient is having an asthma attack and cannot lay supine.

In patients with heart disease, the reaction is more pronounced on the Axillary point on the left side. When I pinch both sides together on such patients, sometimes the skin is thick on the left side only. This is why the Axillary point is valuable as a diagnostic point for heart disease, along with points like CV-17, left BL-15, and left SI-11.

The treatment for coughing or asthma in children under three years of age is simple. Just place an intradermal needle in the Axillary point on the more sensitive side, perform simple insertion (tonification) at LU-9 on one side, and stimulate the upper back with contact needling.

When a patient has intercostal neuralgia, the point that is most tender is often close to the Axillary point. I had one female patient who complained of heaviness and discomfort in the left thoracic region that remained after a cold. Her symptom disappeared with a simple treatment of tonifying LU-9 on the left, needling and direct moxibustion on the induration at BL-13 on the left, and placing an intradermal needle in her left Axillary point.

LU-1 (*chū-fu / zhōng fǔ*)

(SYSTEMATIC): "One unit below LU-2. In the depression three intercostal spaces above the nipple [where] a pulse can be palpated. Locate with the patient supine."

(ILLUSTRATED): "Locate LU-2 in the depression just inferior to the lateral end of the clavicle. Go about one inch below, over the strand of the pectoralis major, to find [this point]."

LOCATION: One unit below the depression just inferior to the lateral end of the clavicle (Fig. 2-44).

PALPATION: Place the tip of the middle finger in the depression just below the

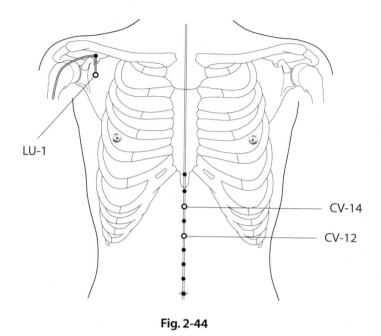

Fig. 2-44

lateral end of the clavicle (medial and inferior to the coracoid process). Move the finger downward while making a back-and-forth movement over the muscle fibers. One goes over many strands of the pectoralis major. Locate the point on the tightest strand of muscle tissue.

INSERTION: Use a vertical, superficial insertion.

INDICATION: Thoracic outlet syndrome, especially hyperabduction syndrome, and also coughing or wheezing when there is an imbalance in the Lung meridian.

DISCUSSION: LU-1 is the front alarm point of the Lung meridian. Front alarm points are used when the meridian imbalance is clear, the pattern has been determined, and there is an organ symptom. I often use alarm points as a set with the associated point of the same meridian. This is how I prefer to use alarm points.

CV-14 *(ko-ketsu / jù què)*   ★★★

(SYSTEMATIC): "It is the alarm point of the Heart. Locate one unit below CV-15."

(*ILLUSTRATED*): "Two units below the inferior end of the sternal body. This is also one unit below CV-15."

LOCATION: Just below the inferior tip of the xiphoid process (Fig. 2-44).

PALPATION: Slide a fingertip down over the tip of the xiphoid process, and look for a tender point. Palpate the point very gently when the area is very tense. Apply a little more pressure when the area is soft, flaccid, or depressed. You can also try pinching the point to see if it is sensitive.

INSERTION: Use a vertical, shallow insertion.

INDICATION: Gastrointestinal disorders, especially stomach problems, heart disease, insomnia, coughing and wheezing.

DISCUSSION: Fullness in the epigastrium (*shinkaman/xīn xià mǎn*) is a condition in which the area around CV-14 becomes hard and there is pain or discomfort when pressed. The term 'fullness in the epigastrium' originally appears in *Discussion of Cold Damage* and was first used in herbal medicine. There are related terms such as 'focal distention in the epigastrium', 'clumping in the epigastrium', 'urgency in the epigastrium', 'hardness in the epigastrium', and 'rock hardness in the epigastrium'. These distinctions were made by subjective and objective sensations of the epigastrium, and different formulas are used for each condition. There is no need to make such distinctions about the quality of the epigastric tension for acupuncture. To obtain the best results, however, one should needle other parts of the body before treating the epigastric area.

When someone has stomach pain and nausea, for example, I first needle a few five-phasic points and points on the head and back. Often this greatly reduces the tension in the epigastric area, which means that the tension was caused by a functional disorder and that the problem did not originate in that immediate area. When needling other points does little to relieve the tension, we can suspect some pathology in the immediate area. In cases like this, it makes sense to needle CV-15 directly.

Asthmatic patients often have tightness between CV-12 and CV-14. Once the five-phasic points are needled and the asthma is relieved and breathing becomes normal, the epigastric area also becomes soft. It is also acceptable to needle points on the abdomen directly. Once I had a bad cough that recurred every night for no apparent reason. While in bed, I inserted a needle in CV-14 and applied rotation for a long time, and finally the coughing stopped completely. CV-14 is also useful for insomnia. I usually have no trouble getting to sleep, but on those rare occasions that

I do, I insert a needle shallowly in CV-12 or CV-14 and apply rotation. I then fall asleep with the needle still in the point. It is interesting to note that insomnia is listed as one of the symptoms for Spleen meridian imbalances in Chapter 10 of *Vital Axis*. It does seem that patients with stomach problems also tend to have problems sleeping.

CV-12 (*chū-kan / zhōng wǎn*)

(*ILLUSTRATED*): "The distance between the bottom of the sternum and the navel is designated as eight units. Locate in the center, four units [from either end] on the linea alba."

LOCATION: At the midpoint between the bottom of the sternum and the navel (Fig. 2-44).

PALPATION: CV-12 is located between CV-11 and CV-13, wherever the reaction is most clear. Often it ends up being a little above the midpoint between the bottom of the sternum and the navel. Press with the tip of the middle finger, adding small circles or a slight back-and-forth motion.

INSERTION: Use a vertical, shallow insertion. Master Miura, my teacher, never inserted needles directly into the linea alba. Instead, he inserted needles diagonally in points slightly off to the side, with the needle angled toward the center. It is actually fine to insert needles vertically into the linea alba. The induration is at a certain depth, and the needle tip simply needs to reach it. When a patient has a surgical scar on the median line, however, it is better to insert needles diagonally from the side.

INDICATION: Gastrointestinal disorders, insomnia.

DISCUSSION: The Spleen and Stomach occupy the central position in the five phases, as well as in the body as a whole. CV-12 is the representative point for the middle burner, which includes the Spleen and Stomach. Stomach qi becomes deficient when digestion is poor. CV-12 is the main diagnostic point for the digestive organs, as well as a major treatment point.

Not long after I opened my practice, a man who lived in the house across the street experienced really bad stomach pain. I therefore paid him a house call. Treating distal points on the arms and legs is my standard practice today, but in those days I went straight to the problem area. So I started right off needling points in the abdomen. After inserting a few needles, the man announced in a loud voice that the pain had worsened. He was having an acute stomach spasm. I tried to compose myself and think of what else to do, but I could not recall which distal points to use. So I asked him where, exactly, the pain was. He pointed right at CV-12 so I gently placed a needle on the point and inserted it with great care. When the needle had penetrated the skin just a few millimeters, the man said "It stopped." I was greatly relieved and then in a flash I recalled points like ST-34 and BL-50. It was at this point that I also remembered what my teacher had told me about stomach spasms, that is, that you should end the treatment as soon as it was relieved, even after just one needle, because it could return with more treatment. So I concluded the treatment. It is strange how needling the same point made the pain worse, only to improve when I needled it again. This is the mystery of acupuncture points, and the thing that makes practicing acupuncture such a challenge.

CV-9 (sui-bun / shuǐ fēn)   ★★

(SYSTEMATIC): "One unit below CV-10; one unit above the navel."

LOCATION: One unit above the navel (Fig. 2-45).

PALPATION: Place the middle finger on the navel and slide it superiorly on the linea alba. Go up to about two finger-widths above the navel, and move the fingertip in small circles to find an induration. Sometimes there is a pulsation, which is not unusual at points around the navel.

INSERTION: A vertical, shallow insertion is most effective.

INDICATION: CV-9 improves the elimination of fluids. Use this point when there is edema or stagnation of fluids and when there is an imbalance in the Kidney meridian.

DISCUSSION: The first serious disease I contracted in my youth was peritonitis, and I remember my teacher needling and applying moxa on points around my navel. He had members of my family apply moxa on these points every day thereafter, and I still recall how hot it was to receive moxibustion by novices on points close to the inflammation. It was every bit as painful as the moxibustion on GB-21 when I got pleuritis.

CV-9 serves as an indicator for the Kidney as well as the Spleen and Stomach. When CV-9 is resilient, the Spleen and Stomach are healthy, and when it is soft just above the navel, the Spleen and Stomach are deficient or injured. The pulse of the

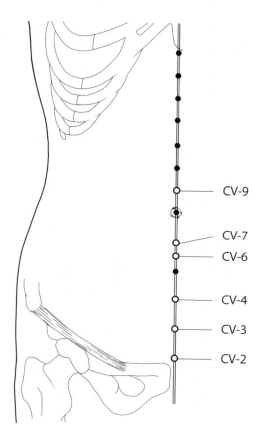

CV-9

CV-7
CV-6

CV-4

CV-3

CV-2

Fig. 2-45

abdominal aorta is very strong at my CV-9. According to one source, it seems that the chronic diarrhea I had during my bout with peritonitis was the cause of this strong pulsation.

People who have a disturbance at this point have previously been afflicted with chronic diarrhea. Also, there is no doubt that CV-9 will be disturbed in those who still suffer from diarrhea to this day. (Taki, 1843)

People who have something wearing on their nerves also have a strong pulsation at CV-9. The most effective way to reduce such pulsation is to needle the five-phasic points on the arms and legs. Thus, points like SP-3 and KI-7 are useful. To treat diarrhea, both of an acute and chronic nature, locate points around the navel with pulsations, such as CV-9, KI-16, and CV-7. Needle these points shallowly, and slowly apply rotation for a long time. This will also relieve the discomfort in the abdomen.

CV-7 (*in-kō / yīn jiāo*)

(SYSTEMATIC): "One unit below the navel."

(ILLUSTRATED): "Designating the distance between the navel and the superior border of the pubic symphysis as five units, locate [this point] one unit below the navel."

LOCATION: One unit below the navel (Fig. 2-45).

PALPATION: Use the same technique as described for CV-9. Stroke the midline downward from the navel, and locate by adding a circular or a back-and-forth motion.

INSERTION: Use a vertical or diagonal shallow insertion, with the needle pointed downward.

INDICATION: Lower back pain, diarrhea, and distention in the lower abdomen. The use of CV-7 is especially effective when there is a Kidney meridian imbalance.

CV-6 (*ki-kai / qì hǎi*)

(SYSTEMATIC): "One-and-a-half units below the navel."

(ILLUSTRATED): "Designating the distance between the navel and the superior border of the pubic symphysis as five units, locate [this point] one-and-a-half units below the navel."

LOCATION: 1.5 units below the navel (Fig. 2-45).

PALPATION: Move the fingertip vertically or horizontally while pressing to locate the reaction.

INSERTION: Use a diagonal and superficial or shallow (5mm) insertion, with the needle pointed downward.

116

INDICATION: Pain in the lower abdomen, especially in the iliocecal region, and for psychosomatic and autonomic disorders. Pathological changes in the right lower abdomen, such as appendicitis, are reflected at CV-6.

DISCUSSION: In Fukaya- and Sawada-style moxibustion, multiple cones of direct moxibustion are applied to CV-6 for appendicitis. If the active point is located precisely, this method works very well indeed. My mother lived with us in her old age. One winter when she was about 80-years old, she woke up with severe abdominal pain in the middle of the night. I found a big lump in the lower right abdomen that was very tender, so I suspected appendicitis. My mother was advanced in age, so rather than send her to the hospital for surgery, I decided to try direct moxibustion on CV-6.

My wife and I took turns applying moxa on the same point for about three hours. I lost count of how many cones we applied, but it must have been several hundred. By the time it started to grow light outside, the pain was completely gone, and after that time, until the day she died at the age of eighty-two, my mother never complained about lower abdominal pain.

CV-4 *(kan-gen / guān yuán)*   ★★★

(BASIC QUESTIONS): "CV-4 is three units below the navel."

(ILLUSTRATED): "Designating the distance between the navel and the superior border of the pubic symphysis as five units, locate [this point] three units below the navel."

LOCATION: Three units below the navel (Fig. 2-45).

PALPATION: Use the same technique as described for CV-6.

INSERTION: Use a diagonal, downward insertion. Shallow insertion sometimes causes a sensation in the genitals. At times, even without trying to do so, the needle goes in quite deeply.

INDICATION: Distention in the lower abdomen, urogenital problems, depression.

DISCUSSION: When it comes to CV-4, CV-5, and CV-6, I do not concern myself with the exact location. Instead, I take all these points together as one area for treatment and select the most reactive point. The reaction ranges from a tight band of tension to a pulsation or a large depression. Any obvious difference, regardless of the nature of the reaction, can be used as the basis for the point location. This is the way that I treat this very important area, which is emphasized in Chapter 8 of *Classic of Difficulties*: "[It is] the source of the qi of life, the root of the meridians, the pulsation between the Kidneys."

It is common for the center of the lower abdomen to be depressed and lacking in strength. When the lower abdomen is weak, the upper abdomen tends to be tight, and the region between CV-12 and CV-14 also becomes hard. If this is the case, I tonify the lower abdomen to draw the qi down. Then the discomfort that the patient had been feeling in the chest and abdomen is mysteriously relieved. This reminds me of a type of abdominal accumulation called 'running piglet', which is discussed in Chapter 56 of *Classic of Difficulties*:

> Accumulations related to the Kidney are called running piglets. They originate in the lower abdomen and go up to the epigastrium. They are like piglets because they go up and down unexpectedly and without ceasing for a long time. Such a person has wheezing and inversion of qi, withering of bones, and shortness of breath.

I see patients with abdomens like this who have heart conditions. Also, be sure to tonify this area thoroughly in patients with depression or autonomic dysfunction who have a soft lower abdomen. Direct moxibustion is good when a patient has a cold condition. Zen meditation and other breathing techniques that emphasize awareness of the lower abdomen aim to strengthen this area. When energy in the lower abdomen is ample, the shoulders relax, the upper body feels light, and the head feels clear.

The lower abdomen naturally becomes soft as a person becomes older. This must be a tendency toward deficiency, but it cannot be called pathological. The lower abdomen of a healthy old person feels evenly soft in both the skin and muscles, so it actually feels nice:

> Old people are prone to deficiency below and excess above. The qi below the navel is weak and the consistency [of the lower abdomen] is soft, while there is tension above the navel to CV-15. This is to be expected with old people. (Taki, 1843)

In the Mubun School, a classical style of acupuncture in which a needle was tapped into abdominal points with a small hammer, acupuncture on points around CV-4 was called the 'fire drawing technique' *(hibiki-no-hari)*. It is stated that this technique keeps pathogenic qi from rising to the head and allows one to live peacefully. It is true that needling around CV-4 is very effective for postpartum depression and mental disorders. The needle, however, does not need to be tapped in with a hammer for this effect. The standard insertion method of using a tube works fine.

It is best, however, if thin needles made of a soft material like silver or gold are used. I once treated a female patient who had started acting strange after giving birth and was going to be institutionalized the next day. After a series of acupuncture treatments, her mental condition improved and she was able to avoid hospitalization.

In some biomedical imaging tests for the kidneys and bladder, a catheter is inserted up the urethra. The insertion of this catheter is extremely painful, and it also injures the urethra, resulting in pain during urination. When I palpate the abdomen of patients who have undergone this procedure, I often find that there is an induration the size of a soybean between CV-4 and CV-5. In such cases I insert a needle gently and shallowly in the induration, and it produces a pleasant sensation in the urethra. Since this condition is an injury rather than a disease as such, the effect of acupuncture is very rapid. Also, once the pain with urination is resolved, the induration around CV-4 disappears as well. It is clear, therefore, that Conception vessel points on the lower abdomen are directly linked to the urogenital viscera.

Once I treated an old woman who had chronic vaginitis that caused pain whenever she walked. She told me that she felt tired for two days after the acupuncture treatments, but that the pain was a little better after that. She was very thin, and I found a groove-like depression in the Conception vessel below the navel. There were no tender points so I inserted a needle very superficially in the deepest part of the depression. I rotated the needle and advanced it very slowly. When it reached a depth of 2 to 3mm, the patient said she could feel a sensation in her vagina. The depth of insertion was so shallow, it really cannot be said that the needle was inserted. It was more like superficial tonification. I needled other points on this patient using the same shallow insertion technique, and I used only a few points. The next day the woman told me that she had no more pain when she walked. It seems that she had been receiving too much treatment. One must be careful when treating old or depleted patients.

In another case, I once had a female patient who had her own business and kept having more children. This was before the advent of birth control pills in Japan, and after her sixth child, she began to get concerned. She was the picture of health, but she wanted me to do something to keep her from getting pregnant again. I therefore tried inserting a needle two to three units into CV-4. I also applied 14 cones of direct moxibustion on CV-5. I gave her this treatment every day for one week. Several weeks later she reported that she had become pregnant again. After 5 months of pregnancy, my patient decided she wanted an abortion, and she asked me if I could do something. For a week, I needled her every day at CV-4, SP-6, and LI-4—all points traditionally forbidden during pregnancy. There was no response, and she ended up giving birth to a healthy boy. Furthermore, the delivery was very smooth; it was an easy birth.

Illustrated Manual of the Acupuncture and Moxibustion Points on the Bronze Figure says that CV-3 cures infertility in women, and *Supplement to Prescriptions Worth A Thousand Gold Pieces* says a woman will become barren when CV-4 is needled. CV-3 and CV-4 are only one unit apart, and so it is hard to believe that one point cures infertility while the other causes it. Ishizaka Sōtetsu (1812) addresses this issue in his book *Concise Discourse on Acupuncture and Moxibustion*: "I have finally come to realize that the ancients did not always tell the truth."

Thus, Ishizaka Sōtetsu was critical of the classics and questioned the validity of forbidden points. His son-in-law, Ishizaka Soukei (1860), quoted the above passage in his book *Special Stories of Acupuncture and Moxibustion*, and in the foreword to the modern edition of this text, Yanagiya Sorei comments as follows:

> If the technique is correct, it is not impossible to prevent pregnancy. This effect cannot be obtained, however, unless the phenomenon of contraction in internal organs appears after needling the infertility points on the lower abdomen. This is why it is said that, if the needling technique is correct, both seeking a child and preventing a child is possible. Thus, it depends on the conditions. One should not say the ancients were ignorant or untruthful.

I remember my teacher telling me about trying to induce abortion with acupuncture. I asked him about his results, and he told me that it did not work for healthy women, but that it worked sometimes for weak women. He added, however, that complications were likely if it worked, and one had to be backed up by a good gynecologist to take care of the patient afterward.

In *The Illustrated Guide to Practical Acupuncture and Moxibustion Points*, Honma Shohaku (1955) observes:

> Traditionally both acupuncture and moxibustion are forbidden at CV-5 in women, and it is said that if this rule is broken, the woman will become infertile for the rest of her life. This, however, does not seem to be true.

This conforms with my own experience. Becoming pregnant is a natural process, and trying to undo a pregnancy goes against nature. Inducing an abortion upsets the balance of yin and yang. The purpose of acupuncture is to restore the balance of yin and yang. When we consider that the basic intention behind acupuncture is to promote health, it makes sense that both the mother and fetus become healthier even when points on the abdomen are needled. I find it hard to believe that one can use acupuncture to induce an abortion or to cause someone to become infertile. It can be said that trying to induce an abortion is the wrong use of acupuncture, and that a normal birth and healthy child naturally come with the right use of acupuncture. This is as it should be.

CV-3 *(chū-kyoku / zhōng jí)*

(SYSTEMATIC): "Four units below the navel."

(ILLUSTRATED): "Designating the distance between the navel and the superior border of the pubic symphysis as five units, locate [this point] four units below the navel, and one unit above CV-2."

LOCATION: One unit above the pubic symphysis (Fig. 2-45).

PALPATION: Palpate the superior margin of the pubic symphysis and press down on it. This is CV-2. Slide your finger superiorly from CV-2 and move it up and down slightly as you press. The tight point or strand is CV-3.

INSERTION: Insert diagonally in a point slightly lateral to the linea alba, pointing the needle in a medial and downward direction. In *Systematic Classic of Acupuncture and Moxibustion* it is said that a needle can be inserted two units, and this suggests that deep insertion is effective at CV-3. In *A Precious Record of Acupuncture and Moxibustion*, a depth of two-thirds of a unit is suggested, and this is sufficient for patients of normal build. A radiating sensation is felt in the urethra at the depth of about half a unit when you use a thin needle. Begin with a superficial insertion and work your way deeper by rotating the needle.

INDICATION: Urinary frequency, pain or discomfort during and after urination due to cystitis or urethritis, vaginal discharge.

DISCUSSION: Once, during the middle of a treatment on a house call for a old woman with hemiplegia, she suddenly said to me, "Sensei, please wait a minute." Then she wriggled off the futon and crawled off to the bathroom. She returned in about ten minutes and told me, "It's terrible because I have to urinate so often. I am just about ready to give up and die." She was taking some medication for this problem, but to no avail. She told me that there was also pus and blood in her urine, and that it was very painful. It was no wonder she was so distraught because the pain and frequency of urination kept her awake at night.

I told her, "Let's treat your cystitis first and work on your hemiplegia later." The pain after urination went away miraculously after the first treatment, and she thanked me by raising her one good hand in a prayer position. I treated her once a week for three years after that, but she recovered from her hemiplegia only to the point where she could walk around the room on her own. The pain with urination never returned after the first treatment, but the frequency of her urination continued to be somewhat greater than normal.

Antibiotics are very effective against bacterial cystitis, but in some cases they are totally ineffective. Also, antibiotics are useless against cystitis that is not caused by a bacterial infection. Acupuncture works quite well for both types of cystitis. An immediate effect can be obtained by targeting indurations at CV-3 and KI-12. For acute or severe cases, needles must be inserted a little deeper to obtain a sensation in the urethra, and they should be retained for ten minutes. Direct moxibustion is also effective. Multiple cones (more than twenty) are advised for acute cases. This is a great method for home treatment. For complete recovery from chronic cystitis, however, I feel that points above CV-3 (somewhere between CV-4 and CV-6) are more effective.

It should be noted that CV-3 is also effective for vaginal discharge. I add this point in the treatment of female patients who complain of this problem, and they are usually pleased with the quick results.

CV-2 (*kyok-kotsu* / *qū gǔ*)

(*SYSTEMATIC*): "Above the pubic bone; one unit below CV-3. On the hairline and in the depression. The place where a pulsation can be palpated."

(*ILLUSTRATED*): "On the superior margin of the pubic symphysis."

LOCATION: On the superior margin of the pubic bone, on the median line (Fig. 2-45).

PALPATION: Press and move the fingertip back and forth horizontally along the superior margin of the pubic bone. Gradually increase the pressure to palpate the linea alba, and locate CV-2 in the small depression within the linea alba.

INSERTION: Use a diagonal, superficial or shallow (1cm) insertion with the needle pointed downward.

INDICATION: The same as those described for CV-3; use the point that is more tender or indurated.

KI-19 (*in-to / yīn dū*)   ★

(SYSTEMATIC): "One unit below KI-20."

(ILLUSTRATED): "It is four units above KI-16, or half a unit to either side of CV-12. This is approximately the midpoint between the bottom of the sternum and the navel."

LOCATION: 0.5 unit lateral to CV-12 (Fig. 2-46).

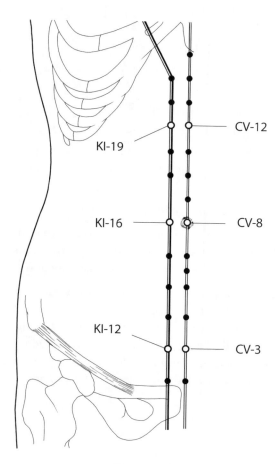

Fig. 2-46

PALPATION: When you find some reaction when stroking over points just next to CV-12, locate KI-19 by pressing and moving the fingertip up and down or in circles.

INSERTION: Use a vertical, shallow insertion.

INDICATION: I use KI-19 as an alternative or supplemental point to CV-12 and ST-21. Therefore, it is good for Spleen and Stomach meridian imbalances and middle burner disorders.

KI-16 (*kō-yu / huāng shū*)   ★★★

(SYSTEMATIC): "Half a unit lateral to the navel."

(ILLUSTRATED): "Half a unit on either side of the center of the navel. Just next to the margin of the umbilicus."

LOCATION: 0.5 unit lateral to the navel (Fig. 2-46).

PALPATION: Place the fingertip in the middle of the navel and move it laterally to the margin of the umbilicus. Go over the margin and move the finger back and forth in line with the Girdle vessel *(tai-myaku/dài mài)* to find a hard or tender point just next to the navel.

INSERTION: Use a vertical, shallow insertion.

INDICATION: Use this point when there is a reaction, and also if there is any indication of an imbalance in the Kidney meridian. By itself, KI-16 is related to fluids, and I use it for loss of fluids, as in diarrhea. I also use it for lower back pain.

DISCUSSION: KI-16 is one of the primary points where a reaction tends to appear on the abdomen with Kidney deficiency. As discussed in my *Japanese Classical Acupuncture: Introduction to Meridian Therapy*, Maruyama Mamoru uses KI-16 and points just above and below it as diagnostic points for Kidney deficiency. Some claim that KI-16 is actually the alarm point for the Kidney meridian. I feel, however, that we should not change the traditional designation of points based on our limited clinical experience.

KI-12 (*dai-kaku / dà hè*)   ★★

(SYSTEMATIC): "One unit below KI-13."

(*ILLUSTRATED*): "Half a unit on either side of CV-3 [four units below the navel]."

LOCATION: 0.5 unit lateral to CV-3 (Fig. 2-46).

PALPATION: Place a finger on CV-2, and then move it one unit above to CV-3. Move it again laterally about one finger-width where there is a strand of muscle that runs vertically. Moving the fingertip back and forth over these fibers, there will be a point that is particularly hard.

INSERTION: Use a diagonal insertion that is pointed either downward or downward and medially at a 45° angle. When a thin needle is inserted slowly and carefully, it will produce a pleasant sensation in the urethra. There will be a strong sensation when a thick needle is used, or when the needle is inserted quickly or deeply. Although this may be good in terms of the effect, it can be very uncomfortable for the patient.

INDICATION: In terms of therapeutic effect, CV-3 and KI-12 are in the same category, but I use KI-12 more often. I use it for diseases of the urogenital organs, pain or discomfort during and after urination, sense of incompleteness after urination, and urinary frequency. I also use KI-12 for turbid urine. I find it useful for problems of the penis, but it does not seem to work as well for problems of the testicles.

ST-19 (*fu-yō / bù róng*)

(*SYSTEMATIC*): "One-and-a-half units lateral to KI-21, on the margin of the ribs on either side."

(*ILLUSTRATED*): "The abdominal points of the Stomach meridian are located three finger-widths on either side of the Conception vessel and are on the rectus abdominis muscle. Palpating with the fingertips, one finds grooves in the muscle and can feel strands of [muscle] fiber. [The point is on a line] in the center between the median line and the midclavicular line. ST-19 is on the upper end of this line, and it corresponds to the inferior margin of the cartilage where the eighth rib attaches to the rib cage. It is about two units lateral to CV-14."

LOCATION: Lateral to CV-14 on the lower margin of the ribs, in the rectus abdominis muscle (Fig. 2-47).

PALPATION: When palpating ST-19 from the left side of the patient, it is more convenient to use the fingers of your left hand. Tenderness and induration can be eas-

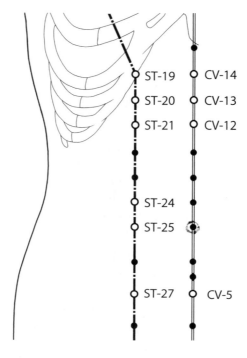

Fig. 2-47

ily detected by palpating lateral to CV-14, pressing just under the rib cage, and adding a small cross-fiber motion. ST-19 is often sensitive to pinching as well. I do not locate ST-19 above the ribs even if it is sensitive. As stated in one of the references above, "It corresponds to the inferior margin of the cartilage where the eighth rib attaches to the rib cage." So I palpate the attachment of the eighth rib and then probe just below that.

Sometimes I do find tenderness above ST-19 between the cartilage of the ribs. I call this Upper ST-19 and sometimes use it as an alternative to ST-19. In the modern text *Acupuncture Point Edition of Illustrated Guide to Oriental Medicine* (Kinoshita & Shiroda , 1985), ST-19 is located in the cartilage of the ribs. The reaction can appear in many places, and sometimes it appears more medially on the lower margin of the rib cage. As a rule, the point that is active is the most effective point to treat. Even so, I do not consider these alternative locations to be ST-19. They are supplemental or alternative points to CV-14 or ST-19.

I like to stand on the right side of the patient and use my right hand to palpate when I want to use ST-19 on the right side only, or when I want to check for gall-bladder disease. I press with my middle finger and add a small up-and-down motion. As I indicated in Chapter 1, when I suspect inflammation in the gallblad-der, I press my fingers in under the ribs and look for a reaction.

INSERTION: Vertical, diagonal, and horizontal insertions are all effective. Superficial insertion is sufficient, but sometimes I go as deep as 5mm. Point the needle laterally when doing diagonal or horizontal insertion.

INDICATION: ST-19 on the right is effective for gallbladder disease. ST-19 on the left is effective for stomach and pancreatic disorders, and for heart disease.

DISCUSSION: In *Concise Discourse on Acupuncture and Moxibustion,* Ishizaka Sōtetsu observes:

> It seems that this point [ST-19] softens spasms in the diaphragm. Needle one-and-a-half units and retain for twenty breaths. Move the left hand ever so slightly, and make the needle move. After needling [this way], the chest and abdomen will feel relieved and comfortable. First check the pulse and, if it is found to be fast, it will be slow after needling [this point]. First check the pulse and, if it is found to be sub-merged, it will be floating after needling [this point]. I have tried this time and again, and I have had this experience time and again.

This passage shows that Ishizaka Sōtetsu was a real clinician. I have had a sim-ilar experience myself. Once, I felt some inexplicable discomfort around ST-19 on the left. I needled the point on myself to a depth of about one unit. I was startled by the sensation when the tip of the needle reached the problem area. It was out of the question to add rotation or lifting and thrusting to the needle at that point. The sen-sation would have been too strong to bear. The key was to move the needle "ever so slightly." The movement of the needle should not even be visible. My technique is to use my right hand for holding the needle, and twist the needle back and forth ever so slightly. This made the sense of discomfort in my chest and abdomen dis-appear.

Tension in the epigastric area is often accompanied by restriction or difficulty in breathing. Relieving epigastric tension with acupuncture effectively removes dis-comfort and tension in the chest and abdomen as well as the back. In the Mubun school text *Compilation of the Secrets of Acupuncture* (Mubunsai, 1685), the area around ST-19 (the Spleen area in the Mubun school) is said to be effective for dis-comfort in the chest and pain in the shoulders. There does seem to be a connection between a stifling sensation in the epigastrium and tension and pain in the upper back and shoulders.

The passage I quoted above from Ishizaka's *Concise Discourse on Acupuncture and Moxibustion* brings up some important issues in treatment. The first one is depth of insertion. I think inserting 1.5 units into ST-19 is much too deep. In my experience, the same results can be obtained with much shallower needling; also, in the interests of safety, I advise insertion of no more than 0.3 unit. The second issue is distal treatment. It is more refreshing and much safer to treat tension in the epigastric area by needling distal points. The third issue is that of local treatment (on the abdomen and elsewhere) and its effect on the pulse. One needle in the right point with the right technique can do wonders. This can also be felt as the 'arrival of qi' and has the same overall effect.

ST-20 (*shō-man / chéng mǎn*)

(*SYSTEMATIC*): "One unit below ST-19."

(*ILLUSTRATED*): "One unit below ST-19. This [point] is next to CV-13."

LOCATION: One unit below ST-19 and two units lateral to CV-13 (Fig. 2-47).

PALPATION: Move the fingertip back and forth vertically or use a small rotation movement to locate the point in the rectus abdominis.

INSERTION: The insertion is the same as for ST-19. I also retain an intradermal needle at this point when the point is reactive and the patient has liver or gallbladder disease (see ST-21).

INDICATION: The same as those for ST-19. Since ST-20 is between ST-19 and ST-21, its indications are a combination of those for these two points.

ST-21 (*ryō-mon / liáng mén*)

(*SYSTEMATIC*): "One unit below ST-20."

LOCATION: One unit below ST-20 and two units lateral to CV-12 (Fig. 2-47).

PALPATION: The same as that for ST-20. Also try pinching the point because sensitivity to pinching often appears at ST-21.

INSERTION: Use a vertical or diagonal, shallow insertion with the needle pointed laterally. Retain an intradermal needle when the patient exhibits sensitivity to pinching.

INDICATION: ST-21 on the right is effective for diseases of the liver and gallbladder as well as the duodenum. ST-21 on the left is effective for problems of the stomach and pancreas. It is also useful for heart disease, discomfort in the abdomen, and shortness of breath (see CV-14). ST-21 is also effective for diseases of the underlying organs, such as the large and small intestines.

DISCUSSION: Sometimes, when there seems to be a problem in the abdomen, no tender point can be found. Yet when I pinch a point, the patient almost jumps with pain. The skin of this sensitive area is thicker than other areas, sometimes up to three times thicker. The pain sensation with pinching is different than that of tenderness. It is often a stinging or burning sensation. Shallow insertion is adequate for points that are sensitive to pinching. Superficial insertion, or just tapping the needle in part way using the tube, is often quite effective.

I think that findings on the abdomen, like sensitivity to pinching, are closely related to stress. No matter what the condition of the patient, I like to needle one or two points on the abdomen if there are reactive points. I find that patients who have sensitivity to pinching on the abdomen are usually under stress and respond well to acupuncture. These reactive points often disappear when the five-phasic points are needled as a root treatment. When I retain an intradermal needle in the abdomen, I target the points with sensitivity to pinching.

ST-24 (*katsu-niku-mon / huá ròu mén*)   ★★★

(SYSTEMATIC): "One unit below ST-23."

LOCATION: One unit below ST-23, and one unit above ST-25 (Fig. 2-47).

PALPATION: Press with the fingertip and move it vertically, horizontally, or in circles to locate a tender point on the rectus abdominis.

INSERTION: Use a vertical, shallow insertion. Retain an intradermal needle if there is sensitivity to pinching.

INDICATION: Duodenal disease.

DISCUSSION: Some patients have stomach pain when their stomach is empty. Often, they have tenderness or indurations at ST-24, and when I pinch the point, it is astonishingly painful. If, in addition to this, pressing the Onodera point (just below the iliac crest on the middle of the gluteus maximus) causes a pain that radiates all the way down to the foot, I suspect a duodenal ulcer. This point was discovered by Onodera Naosuke as a diagnostic point for duodenal ulcers. But even when an ulcer is suspected, a practitioner must be careful with his words. It is not a good idea to declare that there is an ulcer or a problem in the duodenum.

I once had a patient who came in for lower back pain. I found a strong reaction at the above points so I told him there was something wrong with his duodenum. He went to the hospital right away to have it checked out, but tests showed no abnormality. Three months later, however, he had stomach problems and had to have another medical examination. At that time, he had an honest-to-God ulcer. When this patient came in to my clinic months later, he told me that perhaps he was just starting to get the ulcer when I first told him. It takes a medical examination to really determine if there is an ulcer. All we can do is make a guess based on the palpatory findings. Even if there is no ulcer as such, the reactions could indicate a preliminary stage of an ulcer. However, since the body, much as the pulse, changes from minute by minute, such reactions can come and go. Therefore, it is wise to leave the issue vague when warning about the possibility of specific problems. I prefer to advise the patient as follows: "There is something going on in your duodenum. Do not work too hard or stress yourself out. When it gets this way (and I pinch or press ST-24 so they feel how painful it is), the tension always goes to the back and shoulders. It can become an indirect cause of back pain or stiffness in the neck and shoulders."

ST-25 (*ten-sū / tiān shū*)   ★★

(*SYSTEMATIC*): "One-and-a-half units from KI-16. Two units on either side of the navel, in the depression."

(*ILLUSTRATED*): "Two units lateral to the navel. Palpating this point about two finger-widths [from the margin of the navel], there is a groove in the muscle and strands can be felt. This is the meridian. ST-25 is located at the level of the navel."

LOCATION: Two units lateral to the navel, in the middle of the rectus abdominis (Fig. 2-47).

PALPATION: Move the fingertip back and forth or horizontally across the rectus abdominis, which runs vertically.

INSERTION: Use a vertical, shallow insertion.

INDICATION: ST-25 is important as a diagnostic area in abdominal palpation. It is the alarm point of the Large Intestine meridian, and I also use it to determine imbalances of the Liver and Lung when there is a strong pulsation. It is useful to treat this point for intestinal problems.

DISCUSSION: As Ishizaka (1812) says in *Concise Discourse on Acupuncture and Moxibustion*:

> I think all the points from ST-19 to ST-25 can be used to treat various manifestations of abdominal pain. There are three types of abdominal pain. One type is cured by inserting one-fifth to one-third of a unit. Another type is cured by inserting one-half to two-thirds of a unit. And yet another is cured by inserting over one unit. When the disease is shallow but the needling is deep, this causes the pain to get worse. When the disease is deep but the needling is shallow, the pathogen will become even more active. An acupuncturist must carefully determine the depth [of insertion] and be sure to avoid mistreatment.

I refer to Ishizaka's text repeatedly, but this is because it contains a wealth of advice for clinicians. It is different from many other texts on acupuncture points that merely repeat what has been said before by their teachers. It is not easy to bring relief from pain, no matter what the condition. Abdominal pain, especially, is difficult. The insertion can be shallow or deep, but in Ishizaka's case, he seemed to go for the direct method.[7] Although the direct method of local treatment can have a dramatic effect, it contains an element of risk. Hongo Masatoyo, the author of *Precious Record of Acupuncture and Moxibustion*, used the indirect method of distal treatment. In his text, he observes:

> For any type of abdominal pain, doing acupuncture or moxibustion on the abdomen first will actually cause the pain to increase. Be sure to needle points on the legs first and to treat the abdomen only after the pain has subsided. If there is extreme abdominal pain and there is dizziness and a person feels like they are about to die, needle SP-1 and KI-1 to revive the normal qi.

Other points listed for abdominal pain in Hongo's text include BL-60, SP-3, SP-6, and LU-9. Of course, he also recommends using ST-25 right on the abdomen. What can be said from a clinical perspective is that abdominal pain subsides more readily when points on the arms and legs are needled first. Many classical texts suggest indirect or distal treatments, and I believe this is the ideal way.

ST-27 (dai-ko / dà jù)

(SYSTEMATIC): "Two units below ST-25."

LOCATION: Two units below ST-25, one unit below ST-26, and two units lateral to CV-5 (Fig. 2-47).

PALPATION: Locate the point on the rectus abdominis by moving the fingertip back and forth horizontally.

INSERTION: Use a vertical or diagonal, shallow insertion.

INDICATION: Intestinal and urogenital problems.

DISCUSSION: Another passage from Ishizaka's *Concise Discourse on Acupuncture and Moxibustion* notes: "I think that the four points ST-26 and ST-27 cure sterility in men." Ishizaka was referring to hernial or bulging disorders *(senki/shàn qì)*[8] where there is hardness and pain in the lower abdomen. In such cases, Ishizaka thought that "during intercourse the sperm is unable to reach the uterus." For this condition he suggests acupuncture and moxibustion on ST-26 and ST-27. Then, "In time the lower abdomen will become softer. Getting in bed for intercourse thereafter, the dragon's egg will surely be reached."

ST-26 and ST-27 seem to work not only for infertility in men, but in women as well. This same area is targeted with the Chujyo Infertility Moxibustion Point *(Chujyo-ryu fu-nin-no-kyu)* recommended in Fukaya-style moxibustion (Fig. 2-48). These points are all closely associated with the urogenital organs.

LR-14 (ki-mon / qī mén)

(SYSTEMATIC): "The margin of the second rib, one-and-a-half units lateral to ST-19. Directly in line with both nipples above. Raise [the] arms to locate this point."

(CLARIFICATION): "At the level of ST-19 or 20. Each [is] two-and-a-half units [lateral to the median line]."

(ILLUSTRATED): "When moving [the fingers] from the pit of the stomach diagonally down the margin of the rib, there will be a depression where the cartilage of the eighth rib attaches to the rib cage. Locate LR-14 at the lower margin of this [depression]. This is slightly medial to the midclavicular line."

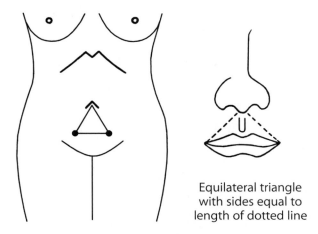

Equilateral triangle
with sides equal to
length of dotted line

Fig. 2-48

LOCATION: Near the medial end of the ninth rib where it attaches to the rib cage (Fig. 2-49).

PALPATION: Find the tip of the eleventh rib, and place the tip of the middle finger on it. Move the index finger medially along the rib cage to find the place where the tenth rib attaches to the rib cage. Next, move the middle finger over to the attachment of the tenth rib, and repeat the above method, using the index finger to find the attachment of the ninth rib. Then move the tip of the middle finger over to where the ninth rib attaches to the rib cage. Move the middle finger back and forth horizontally or diagonally along the margin of the rib cage. To obtain the most accurate location, position yourself on the same side of the patient as the point you are locating, and press the fingertip upward toward the rib cage.

INSERTION: Use a vertical or diagonal, shallow insertion with the needle pointed laterally and superiorly. Intradermal needles are very useful and effective for reactions at LR-14.

INDICATION: LR-14 on the right is used for liver diseases. I use LR-14 when there is an imbalance in the Liver meridian. This point is especially beneficial when there is some dysfunction in the viscera.

DISCUSSION: It is difficult to find tenderness at LR-14. It is especially hard when palpating the abdomen from the right side of the patient. One way is to use all four

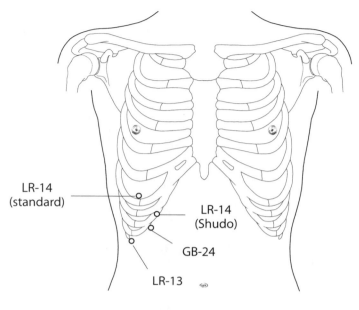

Fig. 2-49

fingers and press superiorly on both sides of the rib cage from below. When patients find this painful, or it feels bad and stifles their breath, there is usually a reaction at LR-14. Also try pressing superiorly into the chest cavity from a point well below the rib cage. In the classics, when the epigastric area as a whole is tight and closed off, the condition is known as 'fullness' or 'stifling sensation in the chest and sides'. For example, "pain under both armpits and extending to the lower abdomen" (*Basic Questions*, Chapter 22). This condition is often listed in the classics as a sign of Liver problems.

LR-14 on the right is used for liver diseases, but sometimes LR-14 on the left is also used. In my experience, when there is liver disease, the reaction tends to appear more medially, closer to ST-19. Thus, I end up using LR-14 less often for liver disease. When there is cirrhosis of the liver, for example, an induration can be palpated in the area below LR-14. This is different from the reaction palpated on the surface or just beneath the skin. Thus, the point of treatment differs from the location of the problem.

Modern texts, like *Acupuncture Point Edition of Illustrated Guide to Oriental Medicine* (Kinoshita, 1985), as well as the Japan Meridian and Points Committee,[9] place LR-14 in the sixth intercostal space. In order to determine which location is better, there should be a study of the reactions at the different locations of LR-14, the frequency of their appearance, and the nature of their clinical effects.

GB-24 (*jitsu-getsu* / *rì yuè*)

(*SUN, 700*): "Half a unit below LR-14."

(*ILLUSTRATED*): "Locate GB-24 slightly medial and about half a unit below LR-14. This is slightly medial to the midclavicular line."

LOCATION: 0.5 unit below LR-14 (Fig. 2-43).

PALPATION: Locate LR-14 where the ninth rib attaches, and move the finger down a little. Move the fingertip back and forth or in small circles.

INSERTION: Use a vertical, shallow insertion.

INDICATION: I use GB-24 on the right for gallbladder diseases. It can also be used in the same way as LR-14 for liver diseases when it is reactive.

LR-13 (*shō-mon* / *zhāng mén*)

(*SYSTEMATIC*): "Lateral to SP-15, level with the navel at the edge of the rib cage. Locate [with the patient] lying on the side with the top leg flexed and the bottom leg extended, and with the [top] arm extended."

(*ILLUSTRATED*): "Press along the rib cage [with the patient] lying on the side, and find the tip of the eleventh rib. Locate [LR-13] just inferior to this."

LOCATION: On the inferior margin of the tip of the eleventh rib (Figs. 2-49 and 2-50).

PALPATION: After finding the tip of the eleventh rib, press a little harder and move the fingertip back and forth in an arc around the tip of the eleventh rib. Also try pressing in under the tip of the rib. Sometimes this point is very tender. It is simpler to have the patient lying in a supine position, both for point location and treatment.

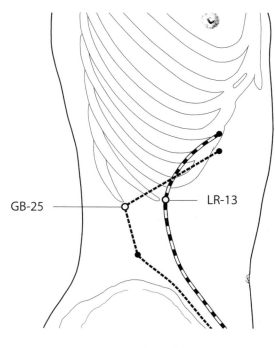

Fig. 2-50

INSERTION: Use a vertical, shallow insertion with the tip pointed slightly medially and superiorly.

INDICATION: Pain in the upper abdomen. I use LR-13 on the right for liver and gallbladder diseases and LR-13 on the left for stomach and pancreatic disorders. I use LR-13 especially when there is pain in the upper abdomen and an imbalance in the Spleen meridian.

DISCUSSION: LR-14 is the alarm point of the Liver, GB-24 is the alarm point of the Gallbladder, and LR-13 is the alarm point of the Spleen. I find it perplexing that these points, which are so close together, each represent a different meridian. When I am in the process of ascertaining the pattern, sometimes I press LR-14 and LR-13 to compare the amount of tenderness. Sometimes there is a clear difference, and sometimes there is not. Pinching these points sometimes reveals more of a difference. Unfortunately, I have not found a satisfactory method of palpating alarm points that consistently serves as an aid to diagnosis.

There is, however, an important diagnostic indicator around LR-13. It is said that a person is likely to have a stroke when the muscles in the flank region of the abdomen are soft and the fingers go right in under the rib cage when pressed. This theory is explained in Yanagiya's *Simple Diagnosis Without Questioning*:

> In those who are prone to strokes, two or three years prior to a stroke, vertical strands of muscle will appear between LR-13 and the anterior superior iliac spine. When a stroke is imminent, these muscle strands will inevitably have a gap where it is mushy and flaccid. When this occurs on the left side, the paralysis will be on the left, and when it is on the right side, the paralysis will be on the right. Now, if the problem is on the right side, it is easy to cure. This is because qi circulates [better on the right side]. Qi does not circulate well on the left side, so these [problems on the left] are hard to cure. Treatment should include qi-circulating and tonifying herbs. When this problem is detected two or three years in advance and treated, a person can avoid a stroke. (Yanagiya, 1976)

The idea of a gap in the muscles around GB-24 where it is mushy and flaccid was peculiar, and it stuck in my mind. I started looking for it after I read this, and sure enough, there were patients who had a marked depression right around GB-24. In several cases, these patients later had a stroke. It therefore seems that Yanagiya's idea is indeed useful for predicting strokes.

According to *Illustrated Guide to Fukaya's Moxibustion Techniques* (Irie, 1980), there are three ways to foretell the likelihood of a stroke. The first is similar to Yanagiya's method. Fukaya has you poke a thumb in GB-24. Normally, there is resistance in the abdominal muscles, but if one side or the other is flaccid and lacks resistance, that is a problem, and that side is likely to become paralyzed. Fukaya had an interesting way of locating GB-24. He would have the patient put his fingertips on his mouth. Fukaya then located GB-24 on the margin of the ribs just under the tip of the patient's elbow.

Fukaya's second method of foretelling a stroke has the patient sit in the *seiza* position. This is the traditional Japanese sitting posture where one sits with the legs folded underneath. Next, the distances from GV-14 and the tips of the acromions are measured to see if there is a difference. If there is a marked difference, Fukaya would consider this a possible sign of an impending stroke, and would apply moxibustion on the shorter side. The points he used to treat this condition are LI-10, LI-11, LI-15, TB-4, and LU-4.

Fukaya's third method has the patient sit on the treatment table with their legs dangling over the edge. He then applied moxa on both M-LE-16 points, also known as the 'inner eye of the knee'. In those with a stroke-prone constitution, this would cause a deep tendon reflex and the leg on the side with the problem would pop up

137

and the moxa cone would fall off. In this case, Fukaya recommended applying five cones of direct moxa on GB-32, GB-39, ST-36, and ST-41.

I have tested all the above-mentioned methods, and they seem to be valid. In the case of the third method, the moxa can be applied on ST-36 instead of M-LE-16. Even when I tell such patients to hold still because the heat sensation will be brief, the heat stimulation causes many involuntary movements in the ankles and toes, which they are unable to stop. And of course, it is easier just to check the patellar tendon reflex with a hammer to see if there is a marked increase on one side.

Yokota Kampū, a contemporary practitioner and author, suggests something that seems to contradict Yanagiya and Fukaya's observations. Yokota noted:

> In my experience, when I do abdominal diagnosis on patients who are about to have a stroke, there is a hardness or muscle contraction on the side of the abdomen which will be affected by paralysis. The extent varies, but for some patients it extends from the epigastrium to the flank region, and for others it extends from the lower abdomen to the flank region. In any case, it is good to keep an eye out for this muscle tension on the side of the abdomen. To treat this condition, there is no need to stick with GB-24. Needle the muscle tension directly. (Yokota, 1995)

Leaving aside the prognosis of strokes, Yanagiya explains his approach to treating the abdomen in *Simple Diagnosis Without Questioning*:

> No matter what the disease, it is important to empty [soften] the epigastric and subcostal regions. Also, acupuncture and moxibustion should be applied on the reactive points on the abdomen regardless of which meridians are deficient or excessive. As to the method for emptying the epigastric and subcostal regions... I will show the approach I routinely use in a figure [Fig. 2-51].

Later, Yanagiya's student Okabe Sodō commented on this approach from the standpoint of meridian therapy:

> This figure means that when there is an abnormality which appears on the abdomen from the Spleen meridian, the Spleen area on the figure should be treated with acupuncture or moxibustion. LR-13 [the alarm point of the Spleen meridian] is also treated along with this. [Likewise] if there is an abnormality in the Lung [meridian], the Lung area is treated with acupuncture or moxibustion. If the [corresponding] alarm points are treated along with this, the epigastric and subcostal regions will surely become softer. This [treatment], however, is given along with treatment of the essential points on the four limbs to balance the meridians. It is not considered sufficient to just needle the abdomen. The needling technique [on the abdomen] should conform to the principles of tonification and dispersion according to the deficiency or excess [state] of the meridians. (Okabe, 1944)

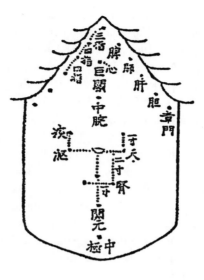

Fig. 2-51

In my opinion, treatment must be given so that, when the subcostal region is tight, it becomes softer, and conversely, when it is soft, it becomes firm. In my experience, the best way to accomplish this is to do a root treatment using the five-phasic points on the arms and legs in addition to needling the tight subcostal region.

GB-25 (*kei-mon / jīng mén*)   ★

(*SYSTEMATIC*): "Below the twelfth rib in the lumbar region, on either side of the spine and 1.8 units below the rib cage."

(*ILLUSTRATED*): "On the inferior margin of the twelfth rib."

LOCATION: On the inferior margin of the twelfth rib (Fig. 2-50).

PALPATION: Probe the tip of the twelfth rib by pressing and circling with the middle finger and by pressing from below in a superior direction. Also, try pinching the point with the thumb and index finger.

INDICATION: Use GB-25 together with BL-23 for Kidney deficiency.

139

DISCUSSION: Studying the location of GB-25 in the classics, some references like the one above from *Systematic Classic of Acupuncture and Moxibustion* (Huang-fu, 259) are not clear at all. In *Compendium of Acupuncture and Moxibustion* (Yang, 1601), GB-25 is placed at the tip of the eleventh rib. In *A Precious Record of Acupuncture and Moxibustion* (Hongō, 1718), GB-25 is just behind LR-13 in a slight depression near the tip of the eleventh rib.[10] Today, it is generally agreed that GB-25 is at the tip of the twelfth rib, but one wonders whether this was the intent in the classics.

GB-25 is the alarm point of the Kidney meridian, but I seldom find a reaction here when patients have Kidney imbalances. This is what may have caused Yoshio Manaka to propose that the alarm point of the Kidney meridian was actually KI-16 (Manaka, 1995). Personally, I have reservations about changing point designations established long ago. Although I seldom find tenderness at GB-25, sometimes when I pinch this point, patients almost jump with pain. The difference in the reaction is very clear when you also pinch other points around BL-52. GB-25 is far more sensitive to pinching when there is a Kidney imbalance. It could be that practitioners in classical times felt for very superficial changes on the skin, rather than looking for deeper reactions such as tenderness or indurations.

POINTS ON THE HAND AND ARM

LU-11 (shō-shō / shào shāng) ★★

(BASIC QUESTIONS): "Medial side of thumb, needle [the point] the width of a leek distant from the corner [of the nail]."

(ILLUSTRATED): "One-tenth of a unit away from the radial side of the base of the thumbnail. Pressing the flesh at the side of the nail and moving [your fingertip] proximally, one runs into the bone of the finger. This is the point."

LOCATION: On the radial side of the thumb, 0.1 unit proximal to the corner of the thumbnail (Fig. 2-52).

PALPATION: The method described above for locating this point in *The Illustrated Manual to Practical Acupuncture and Moxibustion Points* (Honma, 1955) is very good. When you slide the tip of the index finger proximally along the radial aspect of the thumbnail, it runs into a bone. There is a slight depression. Move the fingertip back and forth a little to locate the exact point. Also, to check for tenderness, you can pinch both sides of the base of the nail with your thumb and index finger.

INSERTION: Use a superficial insertion, or prick and bleed a few drops.

INDICATION: Throat pain.

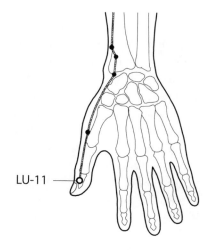

Fig. 2-52

DISCUSSION: Bleeding LU-11 is very effective for throat pain, even in cases of tonsillitis when the patient has a high fever. It is not rare for patients who have been to a hospital and have been on antibiotics for a week to get complete relief after just one treatment. Bleeding by definition is dispersion (draining). Bleeding LU-11 works especially well for cases of Lung deficiency. This may not sound right, but the logic behind it is as follows: In the five phases, when the Lung and Spleen become deficient, the Heart and/or Liver tend to become excessive. In this case LU-10, the spring (fire) point of the Lung meridian, can be needled to disperse the Heart. Also LU-11, the well (wood) point of the Lung meridian, can be needled to disperse the Liver (Fig. 2-53). In practice, both LU-10 and LU-11 are effective points for tonsillitis.

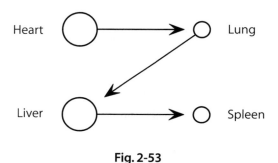

Fig. 2-53

    The method for bleeding LU-11 is to wrap some string around the thumb below the first joint and let it turn red. Then place a thin stainless steel needle and a tube over the point and hit both the tube and the head of the needle diagonally at the same time with some force. This will drive the needle in 1 or 2mm. Remove the tube and needle and squeeze or 'milk' the thumb so it bleeds. There is no need to make it bleed profusely, as just a drop or two will suffice. With some practice, you will not need to wrap a string around the thumb.

    When it comes to bleeding well (wood) points, I recall the brilliant demonstrations of the technique by Maruyama Akio at a meridian therapy seminar. He first checked all the well (wood) points by pinching both sides of the base of each nail with his thumb and index finger. Then he would bleed those points which were reactive or tender by pricking the point with a needle and squeezing or milking the finger. I have tried to emulate Maruyama's technique in my own practice, but I still cannot do it as well as he.

LU-11 is used in Sawada-style moxibustion, along with the point on the opposite corner of the nail, for paronychia (infection on the side of the nail). I find, however, that Fukaya's method of applying moxa directly on the nail, one-third of the way down from the tip (Fig. 2-54), to be quicker and more effective, not to mention less painful. Burning moxa on the affected nail usually does not hurt when a person has paronychia. Moxa cones are burned repeatedly on the nail until the burning sensation is felt.

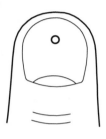

Fig. 2-54

LU-10　(*gyo-sai* / *yú jì*)

(*SYSTEMATIC*): "Behind the main joint of the thumb, on the inside, in the dispersed vessels."

(*ILLUSTRATED*): "Located in the depression distal and medial to the head of the first metacarpal. There are the following views:

1. between the head of the first metacarpal and the trapezium;
2. at the middle of the first metacarpal;
3. in the joint of the first metacarpal and the first proximal phalanx."

LOCATION: At the midpoint between the first metacarpal phalangeal joint and PC-7, in the abductor pollicis brevis muscle (Fig. 2-55).

PALPATION: Press and move the fingertip across the muscle fibers to find the most tender point.

INSERTION: Use a vertical, superficial insertion. Do not retain the needle.

INDICATION: Thumb pain and sore throat from tonsillitis or upper respiratory infections. In cases of 'trigger finger', use the first location described above from

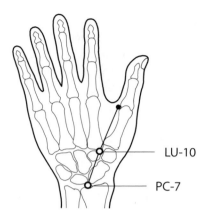

Fig. 2-55

The Illustrated Manual to Practical Acupuncture and Moxibustion Points, which is slightly on the ulnar side of the joint.

LU-9 *(tai-en / tài yuān)*   ★★★

(VITAL AXIS): "One unit above LU-10 in the middle of the depression is the point."

(ILLUSTRATED): "On the transverse crease of the wrist, distal and medial to the styloid process of the radius. Locate in the middle of the pulsation."

LOCATION: On the transverse crease of the wrist in the middle of the pulse (Fig. 2-56).

PALPATION: Gently press with the fingertip and move it back and forth across the radial artery where it intersects the crease of the wrist. Locate LU-9 in the depression. Do not be concerned about the location of the artery when it cannot be palpated where it should be. When that happens, just locate LU-9 in the depression on the radial end of the crease of the wrist.

INSERTION: Use a vertical, superficial insertion. Since this point is directly over the artery, the needle should be inserted no deeper than 1 or 2mm. Do not retain the needle.

INDICATION: I use LU-9 for Lung deficiency when I want to tonify both the Lung

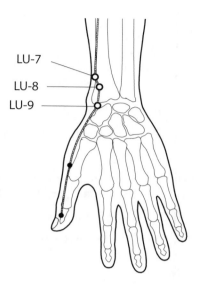

Fig. 2-56

and Spleen meridians. LU-9 is effective for the common cold and coughing, regardless of the pattern.

DISCUSSION: LU-9 is the first five-phasic point I have listed. Five-phasic points, unlike the other points I have been discussing, have special properties. Once I determine the pattern, I consider the tonifying and draining properties of the five-phasic points and treat specific points. As long as the pattern is chosen correctly, the five-phasic points I select work wonders. I feel that their effects are several times greater than that of other points.

In cases of Lung deficiency, often the Spleen meridian, which belongs to the mother phase, is also weak. The Large Intestine meridian, the yang meridian paired with the Lung meridian, is also affected. Lung deficiency, therefore, usually includes symptoms of poor digestion and absorption, as well as dysfunction of the colon. When LU-9 is needled superficially, you often hear abdominal sounds in the iliocecal region (right, lower abdomen), and the patient feels the release of tension in the pit of the stomach. This effect is due to LU-9 being the stream (earth) point.

For the five-phasic points used in the root treatment, it is important to palpate for changes in qi on the surface. Therefore, instead of pressing the point, it is best to stroke the point with your fingertip along the meridian or in small circles. Bear this difference in mind when trying to locate five-phasic points discussed hereafter.

LU-8 *(kei-kyo / jīng qú)*

(VITAL AXIS): "It is in the middle of the *sunkō/cùn kǒu* [radial pulse at the crease of the wrist]. It beats without ceasing."

(SYSTEMATIC): "In the depression."

LOCATION: On the radial artery, proximal to the styloid process of the radius (Fig. 2-56).

PALPATION: Pressing gently with the tip of the middle finger and moving laterally back and forth will reveal the position of the artery. Locate LU-8 directly over the artery.

INSERTION: Use a superficial insertion just deep enough to contact the artery. Just as with LU-9, this point is needled very superficially, as if using a contact needling technique. Do not retain the needle.

INDICATION: Lung deficiency when there is fever or coughing.

DISCUSSION: The landmark for locating LU-8 is the radial eminence of the styloid process. In *Newly Compiled Addition to the Secrets of Pulse Diagnosis,* Manase Dosan observes:

> There is a bone [on the lateral side of the wrist] called the high bone. Do not locate [the middle position] over this bone. After feeling this bone, move the finger toward the proximal position. [Then] press the finger right up against the high bone. Other practitioners say that this [position] is to be found over the high bone, but this is a big mistake. (Manase, 1578)

The radial eminence corresponds to the middle position in six-position pulse diagnosis, but in his text, Manase emphasizes that the middle position is not at the peak of the high bone, but slightly proximal, on the slope of the high bone toward the elbow. Accordingly, LU-8 should be located slightly proximal to the radial eminence (Fig. 2-57).

LU-7 *(rek-ketsu / lìe quē)*

(SYSTEMATIC): "One-and-a-half units from the top of the palm. It separates [here] and connects to the *yang ming* [meridian]."

146

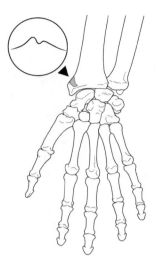

Fig. 2-57

(ILLUSTRATED): "A pulse can be felt between the styloid process of the radius and the tendon of the flexor pollicis longus muscle. [This point] is in this area, one-and-a-half units from the wrist joint."

LOCATION: On the radial artery, 1.5 units proximal to the medial crease of the wrist; about one finger-width proximal to the tip of the styloid process (Fig. 2-56).

PALPATION: Place the tip of the middle finger on the middle position for six-position pulse diagnosis, and then slide it proximally to find a groove. Keep the fingertip in the groove and move it back and forth across the groove. You should find a tender point or an induration. Sometimes the reaction is more proximal than the standard location. This is a point that seems to move quite a bit.

INSERTION: Use a superficial insertion. Sometimes I retain the needle.

INDICATION: Sore throat and pain in the interscapular region.

LU-6 (*kō-sai / kǒng zuì*)

(SYSTEMATIC): "[It is] the accumulating point of the *tai yin* [meridian]; seven units above the palm."

(WANG, 1027): "In the depression, which is like a bowl."

(SHIRODA, 1940): "Master Sawada located this point in the muscle approximately three finger-widths distal to LU-5 and about one unit from LI-10. When there is a reaction, an induration can be palpated. This point often moves up or down, depending on the time and patient. One should find the approximate location and then use the fingertip to locate the most tender or indurated point."

(ILLUSTRATED): "About three finger-widths below the indentation of the elbow one can find the pronator teres muscle, which runs diagonally across the margin of the brachioradialis muscle. Many people will feel tenderness when this point is pressed."

LOCATION: Four finger-widths below the crease in the elbow where LU-5 is located. It is on the brachioradialis muscle (Fig. 2-58).

PALPATION: Place your thumb across the muscle and move the joint of the thumb, that is, the interphalangeal joint, back and forth across the muscle as you work your way distally to find an induration. If you use the tip of your thumb, it is easier to find the point when you press and hold a point as you move the patient's forearm back and forth slightly with your other hand.

INSERTION: Use a diagonal, shallow insertion with the needle pointed laterally.

INDICATION: I use this point when there is an imbalance in the Lung meridian. It is also effective for hemorrhoids.

DISCUSSION: LU-6 is difficult to locate. The reason I say this is because the reaction for this point moves over a large area. It is very effective when it is located

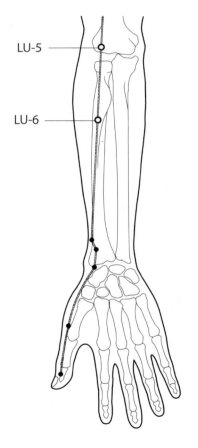

Fig. 2-58

and needled accurately. Occasionally, in cases of hemorrhoids, the needle sensation can be felt in the anus.

It has become generally accepted that connecting points are effective for chronic diseases, and that accumulating points are effective for acute diseases (Honma, 1949). In Japan, however, it was Sawada Ken who first started to associate accumulating points with acute diseases. He said that *geki* (*xì*, the Chinese word for cleft or accumulating) was related to *geki* (*jù*, the Chinese word for severe or violent) (Shiroda, 1940). There is nothing in Chinese dictionaries that relates these two words, so this must have been Sawada's idea. The meaning of the word *geki* for accumulating is a cleft or an opening in the tissue where qi readily collects. I am not sure whether the association of accumulating points with acute diseases came from China to Japan or vice versa, but it says in *Acupuncture and Moxibustion Point Dictionary* that these points "are indicated for acute diseases and acute pain associated with the course of that meridian." (Li, 1986)

Baba Hakkō, an old meridian therapist, said that LU-6 was effective not only for hemorrhoids, but also for bleeding from the lungs (hemoptysis). He was practicing at a time before antibiotics were available, and the only therapy for tuberculosis was rest, fresh air, and good nutrition. This harkens back to the classical age of the *Yellow Emperor's Inner Classic*. It is very rare to see patients in such dire condition come for acupuncture today.

In my youth, I was among the many Japanese who contracted tuberculosis, and I coughed up quite a bit of blood. Master Miura treated me. He probed for an induration between LI-11 and LU-6, and applied direct moxibustion. I still have the scars as a reminder. His point location must have come from Sawada's approach, but I am not certain about the effectiveness of this point for hemoptysis.

LU-5 (*shaku-taku* / *chǐ zé*)

(*VITAL AXIS*): "The pulsation in [the crease of] the elbow."

(*ELABORATION*): "It is [the] water [point]. At the pulsation by the tendon in [the crease of] the elbow."

(*ILLUSTRATED*): "In the middle of the cubital fossa, where a pulsation can be felt. This is where the tendon of the biceps is drawn tightly across the transverse crease. When the medial side is pinched between the thumb and the index finger, there is a slight pain under the tendon. This [reaction] is the meridian, and the point is located here. The insertion must reach under the tendon, so of course the point must be needled diagonally either from the medial or lateral side."

(SHIRODA, 1940): "On the transverse crease [of the elbow] approximately half a unit medial to LI-11."

LOCATION: In the transverse crease of the elbow on the radial side of the tendon of the biceps (Fig. 2-58).

PALPATION: The tendon of the biceps becomes visible when the elbow is flexed a little. There are two ways to find the point:

- *Location A.* A tender point can be found when pressing along the radial side of the tendon with the thumb using a slight back-and-forth motion.
- *Location B.* A hard point or an induration can be found by moving the thumb laterally from the tendon toward LI-11 (Fig. 2-59).

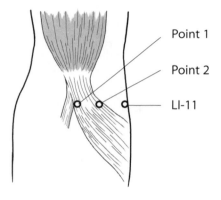

Fig. 2-59

INSERTION: Use a diagonal insertion, pointing the needle in a medial and distal direction.

INDICATION: I use LU-5 for root treatment, especially for Kidney deficiency. LU-5 is the water point within the metal phase, which is the mother of the water phase or the Kidney. Thus, it facilitates the excretion of fluids. For this purpose, I use location A. For symptomatic treatment of throat pain, I use location B.

DISCUSSION: LU-5 is another point that moves around a lot. Indurations tend to appear at location B, but sometimes an induration appears above or below location

B. This location is close to the position for LU-5 in the Sawada style. In any case, the most effective point is the induration. This is a perfect point for home moxibustion treatment for a sore throat. It is best to select points on the arms or legs for home treatment so that patients can apply the moxibustion themselves.

In his text *Kampō Therapy*, Araki Masatane (1957) says that LU-5 is "effective for urinary frequency and nocturnal enuresis." I find that LU-7 and LU-9 are effective for urinary problems, along with LU-5; I often treat urinary problems as Lung deficiency and treat both LU-9 and LU-5. I once got dramatic results for oliguria by doing contact needling at LU-9. These Lung meridian points are also good for cystitis as well as nocturnal enuresis. In cases of Spleen deficiency, I prefer to use SP-3 and SP-9.

The antithesis of oliguria (called hypouresis) is related to the Lungs as well as the Spleen, Kidney, and Triple Burner. When the gathering qi of the Lungs is lacking, the function of straining fluids through the Small Intestine to the Bladder is impaired. This results in frequent and copious urination. People tend to forget this important link between the Lung and Small Intestine in water metabolism.

PC-8　(*rō-kyū / láo gōng*)　　　　　　　　　　★　

(VITAL AXIS): "In the palm, in the space medial to the main bone of the middle finger."

(SYSTEMATIC): "In the middle of the palm, in the pulsation."

(ILLUSTRATED): "At approximately the center of the palm [between the metacarpals of the middle and ring fingers]. In the depression on the transverse crease."

LOCATION: On the palm, between the metacarpals of the third and fourth digit, on the transverse crease known as the 'life line' in palmistry (Fig. 2-60).

PALPATION: Press the space between the metacarpals firmly on the transverse crease, and move the fingertip back and forth in the proximal-distal direction. If there is no tenderness, palpate the points slightly proximal and distal. Tenderness is easy to find, especially when the point is pressed toward the bone.

INSERTION: Use a vertical, shallow insertion. I flick the needle in with force to drive the needle in quickly because this point is very sensitive and superficial needling tends to cause pain.

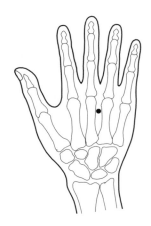

Fig. 2-60

INDICATION: I use PC-8 in cases with palpitations and tightness in the chest when I've decided to treat the Pericardium meridian and there is a reaction at the point.

DISCUSSION: Even though we know that the heart is on the left side of the chest, we are seldom aware of it. Only when something is abnormal do we become aware. Our heart may be beating rapidly or forcefully, or it might even miss a beat now and then. It is a frightening thing when we suddenly become aware of our heart beating abnormally. Sometimes the ECG reading shows no abnormality when we have it checked, and we might resign ourselves to the realization that we are not young anymore.

Most of the elderly women in my neighborhood who I have treated seem to have experienced palpitations at least once. I have gone on house calls where I find family members anxiously gathered around the patient's bed. The patient is holding on fast to her husband's hand. She says "Help! I feel like I am going to die!" Usually the patient is all better before I finish the treatment and begins to laugh with relief.

Just strong finger pressure on PC-8 is often sufficient to relieve a mild case of palpitations or tightness in the chest. The trick is to locate the most tender point. You have to look not only between the metacarpals, but right on the bones as well. At times the tender point appears between the second and third metacarpals. Some texts (e.g., Shanghai, 1977) even place PC-8 between the second and third metacarpals. This actually makes sense when we consider that the flow of the Pericardium meridian goes from PC-7 to the radial side of the nail of the middle finger.

PC-7 (*tai-ryō / dà líng*)

(SYSTEMATIC): "Above the palm; between the tendons."

(ILLUSTRATED): "In between the tendons on the anterior crease of the wrist. Locate between the tendons of the flexor carpi radialis and palmaris longus muscles."

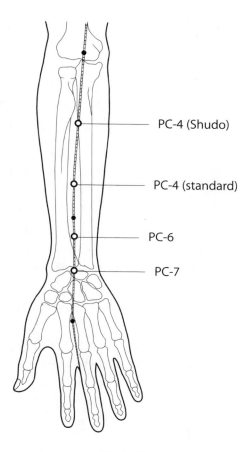

PC-4 (Shudo)

PC-4 (standard)

PC-6

PC-7

Fig. 2-61

LOCATION: On the anterior crease of the wrist between the tendons of the flexor carpi radialis and palmaris longus muscles (Fig. 2-61).

PALPATION: Place the middle or index finger between the tendons above the anterior wrist, and move it down to the wrist. When the finger runs up against bone, move the fingertip back and forth in line with the tendons to locate the point.

INSERTION: Use a vertical, shallow insertion. When the insertion is deep, it can produce a radiating sensation in the palm. This should be avoided.

INDICATION: I use PC-7 along with SP-3 to treat Spleen deficiency patterns. By itself, PC-7 is effective for pain in the wrist when there is inflammation and tenderness.

PC-6 (*nai-kan / nèi guān*)

(*VITAL AXIS*): "Two units from the wrist; it appears between the tendons."

(*ILLUSTRATED*): "Two units above the center of the wrist joint, between the tendons. This is the superior margin of the heads of the radius and ulna, and it is clear how the bones meet."

LOCATION: Two units superior to PC-7 (Fig. 2-61).

PALPATION: Extend the wrist a little, and slide the finger down between the tendons. There is a point where the fingertip catches. There is tenderness when the fingertip is moved back and forth lightly over this point. Do not use excessive pressure.

INSERTION: Use a vertical, shallow insertion. Deep insertion at this point can cause an unnecessarily strong sensation.

INDICATION: Palpitations and digestive problems. PC-6 is the master point of the Yin Linking vessel *(in i myaku/yīn wéi mài),* and sometimes I use it along with SP-4 for extraordinary vessel *(ki-kei/qī jīng bà mài)* treatment.

PC-4 (*geki-mon / xī mén*)

(*SYSTEMATIC*): "Five units from the wrist."

(*ILLUSTRATED*): "Five units superior to the palmar aspect of the wrist joint; it is in the center of the forearm and between the tendons."

LOCATION: On the palmar aspect of the forearm, about halfway between the elbow and the wrist (Fig. 2-61).

PALPATION: Start about one-third the distance from the elbow (PC-3) to the wrist (PC-7) and press the middle of the forearm with the thumb. Work your way down the forearm, pressing points to about halfway down the forearm. PC-4 is in the belly of the muscle. When it appears closer to the elbow, it is in the proximity of LU-6. Also try pinching down the Pericardium meridian to see if there are especially sensitive points.

INSERTION: Use a diagonal, superficial insertion that is angled either distally or radially.

INDICATION: I use PC-4 for imbalances in the Pericardium meridian. Otherwise, I use it for palpitations when there is a reaction at the point.

HT-9 (*shō-shō / shào chōng*)

(*SYSTEMATIC*): "Medial end of the little finger of the hand, the width of a leek distant from the corner of the nail."

LOCATION: On the radial side of the nail of the little finger, 0.1 unit from the corner of the nail (Fig. 2-62).

PALPATION: When you slide the tip of the index finger distally along the medial side of the distal joint of the little finger, it falls into a slight depression between the bone and the nail. Move the fingertip back and forth a little to locate the exact point. Also, to check for tenderness, you can pinch either side of the base of the nail with your thumb and index finger.

INSERTION: Use a simple insertion or bleed a few drops using a No. 3 needle. Thread-like direct moxa is also good.

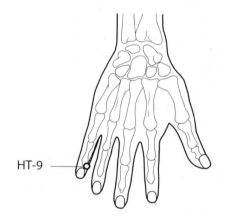

Fig. 2-62

INDICATION: For heart problems, bleed a few drops for emergencies or for acute symptoms. For dizziness or fainting from needle shock, three cones of thread-like moxa is effective.

DISCUSSION: Sometimes, when I am treating patients in the seated position, they will all of a sudden stop talking, take a big yawn, or begin to break out in a cold sweat. Just as I begin to wonder what is going on, they start to faint. I realize they are going into needle shock (vasovagal reaction), and I become alarmed. The patient looks pale, but I must be turning pale as well! There are points I can needle to revive them, such as ST-36, but the fainting was caused by needles in the first place. I am, therefore, reluctant to try another point. As an alternative, I sometimes apply moxibustion at HT-9. This causes abdominal sounds, color returns to the face, and the patient feels much better. Of course, I am greatly relieved as well.

There are other methods of reviving patients, such as massaging their lower abdomen, having them inhale the strong odor of alcohol, or giving them a strong cup of tea to drink. No matter which method you use, it takes a great deal of time and energy to revive a patient once they become faint. Usually, when patients begin to faint, they are in the seated position, but sometimes they are lying prone or supine. I can recall one case of needle shock when needling CV-12, another case needling the lumbar area to treat lower back pain, and two cases needling LR-8. The first two cases were due to excessive stimulation, and the latter two were probably due to mistaking the pattern. In any case, it is better to play it safe and keep the stimulation light.

The well (wood) points are a prime example of points where a little bit of stimulation goes a long way. In Chapter 1 of *Vital Axis* is the passage "The place where [qi] emerges is called the well." The indications for well points are listed for the first time in Chapter 68 of *Classic of Difficulties*: "Well [points] control fullness in the epigastrium." In other words, well points are to be used for patients with fullness in the epigastrium. It is a direct and simple statement. Fullness in the epigastrium means that the epigastric area is hard or tense. This can be subjective or objective, but I find it applies especially when the epigastric area is hard when pressed. Alternatively, the patient can say that they feel sick to the stomach, and the pit of the stomach is tense. There are other symptoms in cases like this, such as severe headache, dizziness, motion sickness, hangover, stiffness in the neck and shoulders, and light-headedness. I have had great success in treating conditions like this using well (wood) points.

Honma Shōhaku writes about the nature of the five-phasic points as follows:

> The place where the water first emerges, as from an underground spring, is called *well*. The place where the water from the well begins to flow is called *spring*. Further, this flow begins to go here and there, and this is called *river*. Where a few of these small rivers converge and form a large river, or join with a larger body of water, it is called *sea*. (Honma, 1965)

Thus, it is generally accepted that the flow of qi and blood through the meridians starts in the same fashion as drops of water coming out of a mountain valley and joining together to eventually form a large river. There are, however, some scholars who disagree with this view. According to Shibasaki Michizō:

The drops of water which emerge from the *well* point remain drops no matter how far they travel. And even if they may be absorbed along the way and disappear, they never become a flowing river. This being the case, the idea that the *well* point is the source of a certain flow is completely wrong. (Shibasaki 1979)

Thus, Shibasaki argues that "the qi which starts at the well point begins and ends at the *well* [point] and does not move on through the spring, stream, river and sea points." (Shibasaki 1979) I am not a scholar, so I just have to speculate from my clinical experience, but a small amount of stimulation at the well point is remarkably effective for fullness in the epigastrium. So I imagine something like vapor moving through a tapered glass tube that is thin on one end and thicker on the other. The vapor is thick and opaque on the thin end, and it thins out to become more transparent on the thick end. When a hole is opened on the thin end (of the well point), the vapor comes streaming out. It seems to me that, the more distal the point, the more dense the qi (Fig. 2-63).

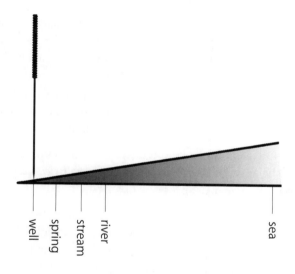

Fig. 2-63

It does not make sense that different parts of the meridians have a quantitative difference in the flow [of qi]. It should be viewed as an issue of density. The meridians are thinner at the tips of the fingers... Viewed from a clinical perspective, being thin does not necessarily mean that there is quantitatively less [qi]. It is actually more sensitive. Comparing this to electricity, it is like a higher voltage... The response to [the] treatment is sharp and rapid. (Honma 1965)

Nevertheless, it seems that Shibasaki agrees that well points function in a similar way when it comes to response to treatment: "The [treatment of] well points... often yields dramatic effects."

HT-7 (*shin-mon / shén mén*)   ★

(SYSTEMATIC): "On the margin of the sharp bone above the palm, in the depression."

(FUKUMOTO, 1986): "On the ulnar end of the palmar crease of the wrist. On the superior margin of the pisiform bone; on the ulnar side of the tendon of the flexor carpi ulnaris muscle."

LOCATION: On the ulnar side of the insertion of the flexor carpi ulnaris muscle on the pisiform bone (Fig. 2-64).

PALPATION: In *The Illustrated Manual to Practical Acupuncture and Moxibustion Points*, Honma states that the Heart meridian passes under the tendon. Pinching and pressing both sides of the tendon with the thumb and index finger, there is a tender place. Honma says the needle can be inserted in this point from either side. I like to use the tip of my thumb to press in under the radial side of the tendon, or to press under the ulnar side of the tendon. When a patient is constipated, I look for a reaction by pressing the pisiform bone distally from the ulnar side of the tendon.

INSERTION: Use a diagonal, superficial insertion on the ulnar side of the tendon, aiming the needle proximally and radially. Use five half-rice-grain-sized cones of direct moxa on the pisiform bone for constipation.

INDICATION: I use PC-7 for the root treatment of Spleen deficiency, and so I seldom use HT-7. I tend to use HT-7 for constipation and apply direct moxibustion on the tender point proximal to the pisiform bone. This use of HT-7 was developed by Sawada Ken, the most famous moxibustion practitioner in modern times.

HT-6 (*in-geki / yīn xī*)   ★

(SYSTEMATIC): "In the middle of the pulse above the palm, one-half unit from the wrist."

(ILLUSTRATED): "On the palmar aspect of the wrist joint, half a unit up from the

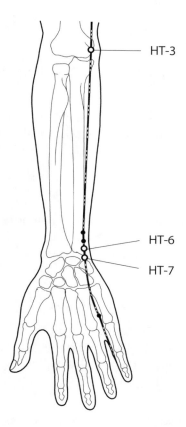

Fig. 2-64

crease at the margin of the pisiform bone. Locate under the tendon. When doing moxibustion, flex the wrist a little to relax the tendon, and apply it on top."

LOCATION: 0.5 unit proximal to HT-7 (Fig. 2-64).

PALPATION: Use the same technique as for HT-7. Press or pinch both sides of the tendon just above HT-7 to find a tender point.

INSERTION: Use a diagonal, superficial insertion on the ulnar side of the tendon, aiming the needle proximally and radially.

INDICATION: Patients with heart problems who experience palpitations or chest pains.

HT-3 (*shō-kai / shào hǎi*)

(*SYSTEMATIC*): "The medial aspect of the elbow, above the joint in the depression. A pulsation can be felt."

(*ILLUSTRATED*): "The ulnar end of the anterior aspect of the elbow joint. It is just anterior to the medial epicondyle of the humerus, on the ulnar end of the crease [in the flexed elbow]."

LOCATION: On the ulnar end of the crease of the elbow when it is flexed (Fig. 2-64).

PALPATION: Place a mark on the medial end of the crease in the elbow, and then extend the elbow. Press around the mark with the first joint of the thumb. Press and move back and forth over the tendons and bone to find a reaction.

INSERTION: Use a vertical insertion.

INDICATION: Tinnitus, baseball elbow, golf elbow.

DISCUSSION: I used to apply moxibustion on HT-3 for tinnitus following the Sawada-style practice that I learned from the text *Basic Study of Acupuncture and Moxibustion Therapy* (Shiroda, 1940). I am still not sure, however, of the effect of HT-3 for tinnitus. More recently I have been using KI-2 as the moxibustion point for tinnitus.

Pitchers in school baseball leagues in Japan are not allowed to throw curves. Straining their arms by overuse, pitchers get medial epicondylitis, the so-called baseball elbow. I use the first joint of my thumb to find the most sensitive point. Often I find that it is more radial than HT-3, and the induration or tender point appears halfway between PC-3 and HT-3. The reaction also appears in the same place for golf elbow. In either case, I apply moxibustion or place an intradermal needle in the point in addition to needling it.

LI-2 (*ji-kan / èr jiān*)

(*SYSTEMATIC*): "Below and medial to the main joint [metacarpalphalangeal joint] of the finger next to the large finger, in the depression."

(*ESSENTIAL POINTS*): "On the radial aspect of the metacarpalphalangeal joint of the second digit, in the depression of the proximal phalanx. The fingertip comes to a stop in this depression when pushing along the radial aspect of the proximal phalanx toward the metacarpalphalangeal joint."

LOCATION: On the radial aspect of the joint between the proximal and middle phalanges (Fig. 2-65).

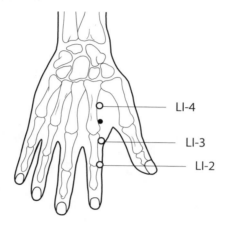

Fig. 2-65

PALPATION: Put a mark on the radial end of the crease in the proximal finger joint when the index finger is flexed. Extend the finger and press and move the tip of the thumb back and forth to find a cleavage. You can also pinch the joint on the radial side with the thumb and index finger and move them back and forth to find the tender point.

INSERTION: Use a vertical, superficial insertion by flicking the side of the insertion tube. To strongly disperse the point, I do quick insertion and withdrawal with a Chinese needle. In this case, I hold the body of the needle close to the tip and poke the point.

INDICATION: LI-2 is a water phase point, and it can be used to disperse the Large Intestine meridian. Apply five half-rice-grain-sized cones of direct moxa for a stye.

DISCUSSION: The Large Intestine, Small Intestine, and Triple Burner meridians have a pair of acupuncture points on either side of the metacarpalphalangeal joint of the arm, and the Spleen, Bladder, and Gallbladder meridians have a pair of acupuncture points on either side of the metatarsalphalangeal joints of the foot. The location of these pairs of points are described in the classics as "the depression below [distal to] the main joint and the depression above [proximal to] the main joint" (see Table 2-1).

Meridian	Below the main joint	Above the main joint
Large Intestine	LI-2	LI-3
Small Intestine	SI-2	SI-3
Triple Burner	TB-2	TB-3
Spleen	SP-2	Sp-3
Bladder	BL-66	BL-65
Gallbladder	GB-43	GB-42

Table 2-1

According to the above definition, the location of LI-2 would be just distal to the metacarpalphalangeal joint and LI-3 would be just proximal. This works fine for root treatment, but for symptomatic treatment, I find that the first location (at the end of the crease) is best.

Before World War II, and for a while thereafter, parents with young children who threw temper tantrums applied moxibustion on LI-2. It served both as punishment and as treatment. So it was a very practical method, but nobody seems to use it today. In the waiting room of my clinic these days, few parents seem to discipline their children who throw a tantrum or scream. Sometimes the father just sits there smiling. They may like to indulge their child, but they do not seem to understand that their child's behavior is an annoyance. Finally, I raise my voice to quiet the child. My wife laughs and says that I am the one who needs acupuncture to calm my temper.

Direct moxibustion on LI-2 is very effective for a stye (an infection and inflammation on the margin of the eyelid). This treatment was known and used by Sawada as well as Fukaya. Pain can be relieved quickly by applying ten cones of direct moxibustion. Even if the inflammation does not subside and surgery becomes necessary, recovery will be speedy and scarring will be minimal. I like to needle Yanagiya's GB-20, along with direct moxibustion on LI-2, to enhance the effect.

LI-4 (gō-koku / hé gǔ)

(SYSTEMATIC): "Between the bones of the hand [metacarpals] of the thumb and the index finger."

(ILLUSTRATED): "In a depression in the dorsal aspect of the hand between the first and second metacarpals. Since the meridian runs along the index finger, it should be located next to the second metacarpal. Probe with the nail to find a muscle fiber that is sore [when pressed]."

LOCATION: Approximately at the midpoint of the radial side of the second metacarpal (Fig. 2-65).

PALPATION: There are two possible locations:

- *Location A.* Press and move the index finger proximally along the radial side of the second metacarpal. There will be a depression about halfway up. There is an induration or tenderness when the tip of the index finger is pressed in under the bone. Most Japanese texts suggest this location.
- *Location B.* Place the index finger on the palmar aspect, and use the tip of the thumb to press the muscle between the first and second metacarpals. Look for an induration. The Chinese texts I have seen suggest using this location (Li, 1986; Zheng, 1983).

Indurations seem to appear more often at location B. I tend to use acupuncture at location A, and moxibustion at location B when there is a strong reaction.

INSERTION: Use a diagonal, superficial insertion that is angled proximally.

INDICATION: Imbalances in the Large Intestine meridian, flushing, neck and shoulder tension.

DISCUSSION: In the days when there were no antibiotics, many cones of direct moxibustion were applied on LI-4 for suppuration, especially infections in the face and upper half of the body. There are marks on the back of my hand also as a reminder of those days. This method was even said to be a way to induce an abortion, but I am not sure about this effect.

In *The Illustrated Manual to Practical Acupuncture and Moxibustion Points*, Honma says that LI-4 is effective for various symptoms of anemia. When I contracted peritonitis as a teenager, I got terrible diarrhea. I had to defecate so often, I finally passed out. When I woke up, I was in bed, and I saw the face of my acupuncture teacher over me. When I asked him later about what he did to revive me, he told me that he had applied strong needle stimulation at LI-4. I also recall a case of infantile convulsions where needling LI-4 worked instantly. The parents of the patient were my next-door neighbors, and they were amazed and grateful.

LI-6 (*hen-reki / piān lì*)   ★

(*SYSTEMATIC*): "Three units above the wrist."

(*ILLUSTRATED*): "On the radial side of the arm, three units above the crease in the wrist. There are two muscles, and the medial and superior one is the abductor pollicis longus muscle. It is the place where there is a strong penetrating sensation when pressed firmly."

LOCATION: On the radial aspect of forearm, three units (about four finger-widths) proximal to LI-5, the base of the first metacarpal (Fig. 2-66).

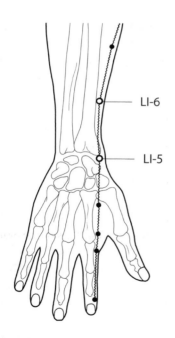

PALPATION: Start from the radial side of the forearm just above the wrist, and press with the distal joint of the thumb as you move proximally. There is a groove between the muscles about four finger-widths from LI-5 where tight muscle fibers can be found. Another method is to hook the thumb and press with the tip of the thumb to move proximally and find a tender point.

INSERTION: Use a vertical, shallow insertion. When there is inflammation, superficial horizontal insertion should be used instead.

INDICATION: Tendinitis, abdominal pain.

DISCUSSION: In Fukuya's moxibustion approach, the thumbs and index fingers are interlaced, and LI-6 is located where

Fig. 2-66

the tip of the middle finger ends on the radial side of the forearm (Fig. 2-67). Direct moxibustion is applied on this point for canker sores and abdominal pain (Fukaya, 1966). This point is distal to the standard location, but it is quite effective when there is a reaction.

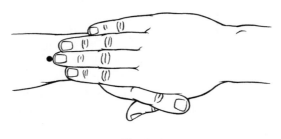

Fig. 2-67

I used to use LI-6 quite a bit for the treatment of tendinitis of the wrist. There are many farmers where I live, and back when they had to transplant the rice seedlings by hand, every year I would see several patients for this occupational tendinitis of the wrist, which is rare today with mechanized farming. Their wrists would swell and become tender. Movement of the wrist also produced a characteristic squeaking sound.

Speaking of the old days, I heard a story about a soldier who got hit by an enemy bullet in battle and grabbed his stomach and doubled over. The pain in his belly was that intense. When he was examined later there was no sign of injury to the abdomen. Finally, they found the bullet wound close to his wrist, in the area of LI-6. This is a story I heard from a patient of my teacher in the 1940s, which for some reason sticks in my mind.

Another episode that I remember in connection with LI-6 is that of a classmate from elementary school who came for treatment in the first few years of my practice. He is the exact opposite of me in that he loves to garden, and that is his only hobby. Furthermore, he does not like acupuncture. I treated him in the seated position for tendinitis of the wrist and he started to feel sick. He got needle shock because I was trying too hard to get results and I had poor technique. He still says he does not like acupuncture, but he comes to me for treatment from time to time. I make a point of using minimal stimulation and keeping the treatment absolutely painless.

LI-10 (*te-san-ri / shǒu sān lǐ*)

(SYSTEMATIC): "Two units below LI-11. Pressing this [point] causes the muscle to bulge. It is on the corner of the straight [brachioradialis] muscle."

(ILLUSTRATED): "Two units below LI-11, where there is a sensation that radiates down toward the middle finger when pressed firmly."

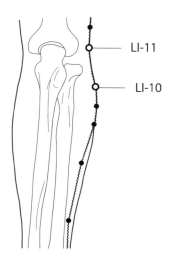

Fig. 2-68

LOCATION: Two units inferior to LI-11 (Fig. 2-68).

PALPATION: Use the same technique as described for LI-6, and press distally along the meridian from LI-11. There will be an induration in the belly of the brachioradialis muscle. I consider LI-8, LI-9, and LI-10 to be one zone for treatment; needle the point that shows the greatest reaction.

INSERTION: Use a vertical, shallow insertion. Direct moxibustion is also effective.

INDICATION: Flushing in the face and neck, shoulder tension.

LI-11 (*kyoku-chi / qū chí*)

(SYSTEMATIC): "On the lateral epicondyle of the elbow, between the bones of the elbow. Locate with the [patient's] hand on the chest."

(ESSENTIAL POINTS): "The lateral anterior aspect of the lateral epicondyle, on the lateral end of the cubital crease."

LOCATION: At the lateral end of the cubital crease (Fig. 2-68).

PALPATION: With the elbow fully flexed, press or mark the point at the lateral end of the crease in the elbow. Extend the elbow and locate an induration or tender point by moving the bone of the distal joint of the thumb back and forth over the point. Sometimes the induration is deep and hard to find. If you have difficulty finding a reaction, hook your thumb and dig in with the tip. Once you become proficient at locating LI-11, it is not necessary to flex the elbow to begin locating the point.

INSERTION: Use a vertical, shallow insertion with the arm extended. To insert the needle deeper, in toward the joint, insert vertically into the end point of the crease with the elbow flexed.

INDICATION: I use LI-11 primarily for root treatment as the tonification point of the Large Intestine meridian. Treating LI-11 has many uses for symptomatic treatment, but its main effect can be summarized as that of drawing qi down from the head. Therefore, LI-11 is a good point for reducing flushing in the face. Deeper insertion is used for pathology of the elbow joint.

DISCUSSION: LI-11 is one of the most important points among the standard treatment points of the Sawada style. LI-11 is used for problems in the upper limbs, while ST-36 is used for problems in the lower limbs. LI-11 is one of the most useful points in moxibustion therapy for regulating blood pressure, as well as for improving health in general.

LI-11 is also important in root treatment. Tonifying the Large Intestine meridian is a way of drawing qi away from the Lung meridian to treat Liver deficiency.

TB-3 (*chū-sho / zhōng zhǔ*)

(*SYSTEMATIC*): "Above the main joint [metacarpalphalangeal joint] of the finger next to the little finger, in the depression."

(*ILLUSTRATED*): "Proximal to the space between the fourth and fifth metacarpalphalangeal joints. In the depression between the metacarpals, one unit from TB-2 [which is just distal to the metacarpalphalangeal joints]."

LOCATION: On the back of the hand, just proximal and ulnar to the fourth metacarpalphalangeal joint, on the margin of the metacarpal (Fig. 2-69).

PALPATION: Press between the metacarpalphalangeal joints in a distal to proximal direction, and you will go over a tendon into a depression proximal to the joint. You can also slide the fingertip distally along the ulnar side of the fourth metacarpal

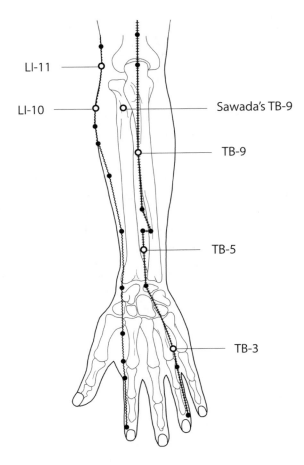

Fig. 2-69

toward the finger until it comes to a stop in the same depression. Press and move the fingertip back and forth along the bone to find a tender point. You might also try pressing in under the fourth metacarpal.

INSERTION: Use a vertical, superficial insertion.

INDICATION: TB-3 is a wood phase point, and I use it to tonify the Triple Burner meridian, which is of the fire phase. Otherwise, TB-3 is effective for the symptoms of dizziness and tinnitus when they are related to the Triple Burner meridian.

TB-5 (*gai-kan / wài guān*)

(SYSTEMATIC): "Two units above the wrist, in the depression."

(ILLUSTRATED): "Two units proximal to the midpoint of the back of the wrist."

LOCATION: Two units proximal to TB-4 (the center of the dorsal aspect of the wrist), approximately three finger-widths above the wrist, between the radius and the ulna (Fig. 2-69).

PALPATION: A depression can be found above the bones when the fingertip is moved from TB-4 toward the elbow. Move the fingertip back and forth slightly in line with the bones to find a tight strand or tender point.

INSERTION: Use a vertical, shallow insertion.

INDICATION: TB-5 is a connecting point so I use it to tonify or disperse the Triple Burner meridian. Also, I give TB-5 a try when there is wrist pain and the focus of the pain is unclear.

TB-9 (*shi-toku / sì dú*)

(SYSTEMATIC): "Five units below the elbow, in the depression on the posterior aspect [of the forearm]."

(ILLUSTRATED): "On the posterior aspect of the forearm. The distance between the elbow and wrist is designated as ten units. [This point] is five units inferior to the tip of the elbow, and is between the ulna and radius."

(SHIRODA, 1940): "Master Sawada located this point differently, two units below the elbow joint. Thus, LU-6, LI-10, and TB-9 line up all in a row. TB-9 is found in the depression in the muscle on the ulnar side of LI-10."

LOCATION: On the ulnar side of LI-10 in the brachioradialis muscle (Fig. 2-69).

PALPATION: I use Sawada's location. First, use the thumb to locate LI-10, three finger-widths below LI-11 (the end of the transverse crease of the elbow). Then move the thumb laterally over the muscle fibers. The reaction is clearly evident when the tip of the thumb is moved back and forth in a cross-fiber motion. It is easier, however, to locate indurations at LU-5, LI-10, and TB-9 by rolling the distal joint of the thumb across the muscle fibers.

INSERTION: Use a vertical or diagonal, superficial insertion. Insert straight in the groove in the muscle, or diagonally as if going underneath the muscle.

INDICATION: Pain and tension in the neck, shoulder, interscapular region, or arm.

SI-1 (shō-taku / shào zé) ★★

(SYSTEMATIC): "The corner of the little finger, one-tenth of a unit from the lateral side of the base of the nail, in the depression."

(ILLUSTRATED): "On the ulnar end of the little finger in the depression, one-tenth of a unit lateral to the base of the nail. Pressing the flesh at the side of the nail and moving [your fingertip] proximally, one runs into the bone of the finger. This is the point."

LOCATION: On the ulnar side of the little finger, 0.1 unit proximal to the corner of the nail (Fig. 2-70).

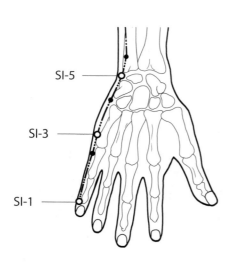

Fig. 2-70

PALPATION: Use the same technique as described for LU-11. When you slide the tip of the index finger proximally along the side of the nail, it runs into a bone. There is a slight depression before the bone. Move the fingertip back and forth a little to locate the exact point.

INSERTION: Contact needling is effective. For painless superficial insertion, flick the side of the needle and tube with a little force. Bleed if there is heat or pain in the Small Intestine meridian.

INDICATION: Discomfort or pain in the chest. I prick SI-1 and squeeze out a few drops of blood when there is pain or heat in the Small Intestine meridian.

170

SI-3 (kō-kei / hòu xī)

(SYSTEMATIC): "Lateral to [the base of] the little finger, above the main joint, in the depression."

(ILLUSTRATED): "At the ulnar tip of the transverse crease of the metacarpalphalangeal joint. It is a point where there is a penetrating pain when pressed hard with the nail. *Systematic Classic on Acupuncture and Moxibustion* says [SI-3] is in the depression above the main joint [metacarpalphalangeal joint]. So, traditionally, it was located proximal to the protuberance of the head of the metacarpal."

(SHIRODA, 1940): "In the depression proximal to the fifth metacarpalphalangeal joint. Located in the depression next to the tip of the transverse crease of the palm when making a fist. In many cases, the tip of the crease itself is where the point is found."

(ESSENTIAL POINTS): "In the depression before the metacarpalphalangeal joint, where the finger comes to a stop when stroking distally down the ulnar side of the fifth metacarpal."

LOCATION: In the depression proximal to the fifth metacarpalphalangeal joint. This is the depression above the main joint mentioned in the classics. Thus, I use the traditional location for SI-3 (Fig. 2-70).

PALPATION: Stoking distally down the ulnar side of the fifth metacarpal, you run into a bony protuberance. A tender point can be found by placing the index finger at a right angle to the skin and moving it back and forth across the muscle fibers, which run parallel to the bone. It is also possible to place a mark on the end of the transverse crease that forms when making a fist. Open the hand to probe above and below the mark.

INSERTION: Use a vertical, superficial insertion. When the skin of the hands is very thick, as in the case of laborers, the needle must be inserted skillfully or it can be very painful.

INDICATION: I use SI-3 to disperse excess in the Small Intestine meridian. I also use this point for headaches, pain in the neck, shoulders, interscapular area, and lower back pain. SI-3 is a master point that is coupled with BL-62 in Extraordinary vessel treatments. Sometimes I use SI-3 as a pair with BL-62 for neck pain, but usually I use SI-3 by itself.

DISCUSSION: According to Honma's *The Illustrated Manual to Practical Acupuncture and Moxibustion Points*, SI-3 is in the middle of the metacarpalphalangeal joint (Fig. 2-71). Personally, I find that the classical location, above the main joint, works better. As explained under LI-2, the classics locate pairs of points above and below the main joint of the three yang meridians of the arm. In this scheme, the point just distal to the metacarpalphalangeal joint is SI-2, and the point proximal is SI-3. Even though I use SI-3 to disperse the Small Intestine meridian, I find that it is effective in alleviating occipital headaches and neck pain regardless of the meridians involved, and so I use it often.

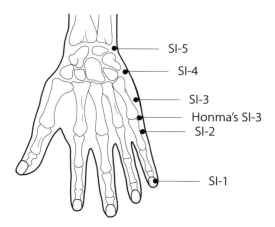

Fig. 2-71

POINTS ON THE
LEG AND FOOT

SP-1 (*in-paku / yīn bái*) ★★

(SYSTEMATIC): "On the tip of the big toe, the width of a leek distant from the medial side of the nail."

(ILLUSTRATED): "One-tenth of a unit from the medial end of the base of the nail of the big toe."

LOCATION: On the medial aspect of the big toe, 0.1 unit proximal to the corner of the nail (Fig. 2-72).

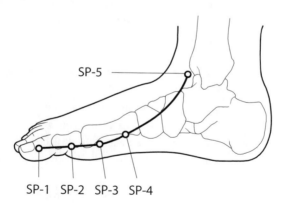

SP-5

SP-1 SP-2 SP-3 SP-4

Fig. 2-72

PALPATION: Contact needling is most effective. For painless superficial insertion, flick the side of the needle and tube with a little force.

INSERTION: Use a vertical, superficial insertion. Perform either simple insertion with some rotation or retain the needle. A tube is not necessary for needling this point. If you use a tube, flick the tube and the head of the needle at the same time to reduce the pain. The needle cannot be inserted very deeply at this point; it will therefore lay on its side when it is retained.

INDICATION: I use SP-1 for gastrointestinal problems with pain. Honma's *The Illustrated Manual to Practical Acupuncture and Moxibustion Points* recommends using SP-1 for mental illness.

DISCUSSION: As previously discussed, according to Chapter 68 of *Classic of Difficulties*, well (wood) points are indicated for distention in the epigastrium. Therefore, SP-1 is useful when there is an imbalance in the Spleen meridian and whenever the epigastrium is tense or hard. I have used SP-1 faithfully in this manner for many years, believing what is written in the *Classic of Difficulties*. Unlike with LR-1, however, I did not have any experience that clearly substantiated this effect. Recently, I had two experiences with SP-1 that justified my belief.

I must have an allergic constitution because, since my youth, there have been things I could not stomach. I could not drink milk or eat much shellfish. There were a few varieties of shellfish that I could eat, but if I ate even a morsel of the others, I got stomach pain and diarrhea a few hours later. As I have gotten older, however, these food sensitivities have diminished, and I can now drink a little milk or eat fried oysters without adverse effects. Recently, a patient gave me a New Year's gift of fresh oysters. Thinking that it would no longer hurt me, I fried them one evening and ate them as a snack with sake. Late that night, about 2 A.M., I woke up with pain in my abdomen. Both my upper and lower abdomen were distended and sore. Soon I got abdominal cramps and diarrhea. Being too tired to stay up, I gave myself acupuncture in bed, placing 40mm, No. 0 needles in SP-1 on both sides. Soon I felt some movement below my navel, and my stomach pain began to ease, as if a tide were receding. The movement in my abdomen subsided, and then the discomfort in my abdomen became localized in the epigastrium. I placed one more needle in PC-7 on my left wrist to take care of this. The discomfort began to disappear, and soon I fell fast asleep.

The other experience I had was at a monthly study group of local acupuncturists, which I lead. Once a participant curled up on his side with a dizzy spell. I tend to treat all cases of dizziness as Liver deficiency, and I placed needles in the standard points for dizziness, that is, LR-1 and the auricular vertigo points. When I checked the pulses after retaining these needles, however, I found that the Spleen position seemed to be quite weak as well. So I removed the needles from LR-1 and placed some in SP-1 instead. That did the trick, and the symptoms resolved right away.

Back when I was a student, Yanagiya Sorei came to visit my teacher's place in Kyushu and gave some treatments. I observed him treat a patient with mental illness. I especially recall how the patient winced at the pain of having his big toes needled. It could have been LR-1 or SP-1, but I think it must have been SP-1.

In his lectures on the *Classic of Difficulties*, Inoue Keiri said that mental illness was usually Spleen deficiency and that the needles must be shallow. He said that just contact needling is sufficient, and the patient will show improvement after a good night's sleep.

I find that contact needling of SP-1 is best for the treatment of elderly patients with insomnia or depression. I once had a 70-year-old man come to my clinic complaining of insomnia. He told me that acupuncture treatments at other clinics left him even more wide-awake at night. I gave him a treatment, taking care to insert the needles very shallowly, and retained just a few. He returned a few days later to tell me that he was still not getting any sleep. On top of that, he told me he did not want any needles in his head or in the back of his neck. I didn't like being told this, but what could I say? It was a fact that the last treatment did not help him. Under those circumstances, I backed way off and did only contact needling, without inserting any needles. A few days later he came back to report that he got one good night's sleep after the treatment, but that the effect did not last. He demanded that this time I give him a treatment that lasted longer. As hard to please as he was, the old man kept coming back for more treatments, and he was in better humor each time, as his sleep progressively improved. He then had the nerve to tell me that I could start giving him "regular acupuncture," like the rest of my patients. Some people!

SP-2 (*dai-to / dà dū*)

(*VITAL AXIS*): "Behind and below the main joint, in the middle of the depression."

(*ILLUSTRATED*): "The first metatarsal and the first [proximal] phalanx forms a large round mound. When the big toe is flexed, a crease forms on its medial aspect near the joint. [The point is] just proximal [to this crease]. The difference between the skin of the top of the foot and that of the sole is visible. SP-2 is at the border, that is, between 'the red and white flesh'."

LOCATION: In the depression on the medial aspect of the metatarsophalangeal joint (Fig. 2-72).

PALPATION: There is a depression where the finger comes to a stop when stroking the medial side of the big toe proximally toward the metatarsophalangeal joint. A tender point can be located by pressing the finger vertically into the point and moving it back and forth.

INSERTION: Use a vertical, superficial insertion.

INDICATION: Stomach pain, gout.

DISCUSSION: Generally, SP-2 is located in the depression distal to the metatarsophalangeal joint. The location given by Honma in *The Illustrated Manual to Practical Acupuncture and Moxibustion Points* is close to the center of the metatarsophalangeal joint. I have discussed in connection with LI-2 how many distal points are positioned on either end of the main joint in the classics. I use Honma's location because it seems to give better clinical results.

SP-3 (tai-haku / tài bái) ★★★

(VITAL AXIS): "Below the joint of the big toe."

(CLASSIFICATION): "On the border of the red and white flesh."

(SYSTEMATIC): "On the inside of the foot in the middle of the depression below the joint of the big toe."

(ILLUSTRATED): "Posterior to the protuberance of the first metatarsophalangeal joint, on the border of the red and white flesh; the place where the finger comes to a stop when stroking the medial side of the first metatarsal distally toward the toe."

LOCATION: In the depression proximal to the medial side of the first metatarsophalangeal joint (Fig. 2-72).

PALPATION: Stroke in the opposite direction from that given for SP-2. The finger will come to a stop when stroking from SP-4 toward the mound of the metatarsophalangeal joint. Pressing often reveals a tender point on the edge of the bone. To locate SP-3 for root treatment, stroke lightly with your fingertip and find the deepest depression.

INSERTION: Use a vertical, superficial insertion. For root treatment or on sensitive patients, use contact needling with the needle tip pointed proximally.

INDICATION: SP-3 is a principal tonification point for the treatment of Spleen deficiency and Lung deficiency patterns. It is also effective for gastrointestinal diseases, abdominal pain, heart disease, anorexia, insomnia, and lassitude.

I also use SP-3 for cases of lower back pain caused by kidney stones. Most cases of acute lower back pain from stones becoming lodged in the urethra have a Spleen deficiency presentation. When the excruciating pain from a kidney stone causes a patient to curl up on the side, I needle SP-3 on the bottom leg. This is usually the unaffected side. The trick is to start the needle without the tube. Even if the tube is used, it is best not to tap the needle in. Just place the needle and tube on the point, hold the needle in place and remove the tube, and rotate the needle on the skin surface. A few minutes of this will relieve the pain.

SP-4 (kō-son / gōng sūn)

(*VITAL AXIS*): "One unit distant from the back of the main joint."

(*ILLUSTRATED*): "One unit posterior to SP-3. The place where the finger comes to a stop when stroking proximally along the [metatarsal] bone from SP-3."

LOCATION: On the medial aspect of the first metatarsal where the finger comes to a stop when stroking proximally from SP-3 (Fig. 2-72).

PALPATION: The finger comes to a stop at SP-3 when the first metatarsal is stroked distally. SP-4 is the depression that the finger gets caught in when stroking proximally. If it doesn't feel like much of a depression, slide the finger down toward the sole to the bulge of a small muscle. This is the abductor hallucis muscle. You can locate the point on this muscle.

INSERTION: Use a vertical or diagonal, superficial insertion with the needle pointed proximally.

INDICATION: Gastrointestinal diseases; I use SP-4 on the left side for constipation.

SP-5 (shō-kyū / shāng qiū)

(*VITAL AXIS*): "Below the medial malleolus, in the middle of the depression."

(*SYSTEMATIC*): "Below the medial malleolus, in the middle of the depression, slightly in front. In the bowl-like depression in front of the medial malleolus."

(ILLUSTRATED): "In the depression on the anterior and inferior corner of the medial malleolus. It is located between the medial malleolus and the navicular bone."

LOCATION: Between the medial malleolus and the navicular bone (Fig. 2-72).

PALPATION: There is a big depression between the medial malleolus and the navicular bone. Place the finger vertically in this depression and work the fingertip back and forth toward the top of the foot (LR-4). There will be a tender or indurated point.

INSERTION: Use a vertical, shallow insertion.

INDICATION: Use for coughing, wheezing, and fever when there is a Spleen meridian imbalance. SP-5 is the metal point of the Spleen meridian, so it can be used as an alternate tonification point for the Spleen meridian in cases of Lung deficiency or respiratory problems. Also, SP-5 can be used instead of SP-3 if needling SP-3 is too painful.

DISCUSSION: There is a great deal about moxibustion therapy in Chikuta Takichi's *Secrets of Practical Nursing Care in the Home,* and I learned much from this book during my convalescence as a young man. Chikuta recommends direct moxibustion on SP-5 for anal prolapse. The first person I treated for anal prolapse was an old lady, and the prolapsed anus, the size of a ping-pong ball, could be felt on the right side through her clothes. She had tried pushing it back in, but it wouldn't go. I do not remember whether I treated her for Liver deficiency or Lung deficiency, but I placed four needles in two tonification points on each side. For the symptomatic treatment, I needled CV-3 and some points on her sacrum. I then applied direct moxibustion on SP-5. In about an hour, the prolapsed anus returned to normal. The prolapse recurred a couple more times for this patient before she finally passed away, but each time, the same treatment corrected it. I am not sure how much the moxibustion on SP-5 had to do with the effect, but it makes sense that a Spleen meridian point would work.

SP-6 *(san-inkō / sān yīn jiāo)*

(SYSTEMATIC): "Three units above the medial malleolus, in the depression beneath the bone."

(ILLUSTRATED): "About three finger-widths above the medial malleolus, and one strand of muscle away from the posterior margin of the tibia. In other words, it is in the tibialis posterior muscle about 0.3 units from the tibia."

LOCATION: Three units above the medial malleolus (Fig. 2-73).

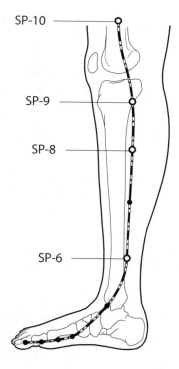

SP-10

SP-9

SP-8

SP-6

Fig. 2-73

PALPATION: You can get a rough idea of the location by finding the point either three finger-widths above the top of the medial malleolus, or four finger-widths above the middle of the medial malleolus. It is best to stand at the foot of the patient and use the distal joint of the thumbs to palpate both sides at once. Roll across the posterior margins of both tibias. When there is a reaction, you will find a mushy or tender point. When all you feel is the margin of the bone, you can assume there is no reaction. You can also use the tip of your middle finger to find depressions by moving the finger in small circles or vertically along the bone.

In *The Illustrated Manual to Practical Acupuncture and Moxibustion Points*, Honma observes:

> The Spleen meridian generally goes along the [posterior] margin of the tibia, but since SP-6 is the place where the Spleen, Kidney, and Liver meridians converge, the point is located slightly posterior [to the bone].

This is one opinion. In practice, however, the reaction almost always appears on the margin of the tibia, and the effect is better when the reactive point is treated.

INSERTION: Use a vertical or diagonal, shallow insertion, with needle pointed superiorly. Retain an intradermal needle or prescribe direct moxibustion at home for gynecological problems.

INDICATION: Menstrual irregularity, menstrual pain, discomfort before and after menstruation, fetal malpresentation.

DISCUSSION: There are few points as important as SP-6 that are not five-phasic points, especially for the purpose of diagnosis. No wonder it is known also as the ST-36 for women. When I palpate female patients, I always check SP-6 because it serves as a diagnostic point for gynecological problems. As for treatment, I recommend direct moxibustion at home. If the patient does not like moxibustion, I retain an intradermal needle. When it comes to acupuncture, however, I tend to use points like SP-3 and Sp-9 instead of SP-6.

SP-6 has been designated as a forbidden point in pregnant women. This apparently comes from the classic *Illustrated Manual of the Acupuncture and Moxibustion Points on the Bronze Figure* (Wang, 1027; Maruyama, 1977), and is based on a story where a prince of the Song Dynasty saw a pregnant woman and conjectured that she would give birth to a girl. However, his minister, Xu Wenbo, took a look and said she was bearing one boy and one girl. Overtaken by curiosity, the prince wanted to find out right away by having her belly opened, whereupon: "The minister said, acupuncture [will do] this if SP-6 of the leg is dispersed and LI-4 of the hand *yang ming* is tonified." The treatment worked, and the babies came out right away. As Xu Wenbo had predicted, there was one boy and one girl. Anyway, it has been said that ever since, SP-6 must not be needled in pregnant women.

In his text *Concise Discourse on Acupuncture and Moxibustion,* Ishizaka quotes the passage about SP-6 from the classics: "Must not be needled when pregnant. Will cause an abortion every time." He follows this with the comment, "[It is said that] people in ancient times had this experience. I do not believe it to be true."

Previously, in my discussion of CV-4, I mentioned how I tried to induce abortion with acupuncture without any success. Nevertheless, it is not a good idea to needle SP-6 deeply on pregnant women. I have heard of acupuncture treatments causing an abortion, and even if a person is not pregnant, it is obvious that needling carelessly, excessively deep, or using big needles can injure a patient. Ever since I started practicing meridian therapy, my acupuncture has become more precise, my insertions more shallow, and I use thinner needles. Treatments like this have a beneficial effect on both the pregnant mother and the fetus, and the child is almost certain to like acupuncture. This is prenatal education about acupuncture. There are many pregnant women who become ill and are worried about taking drugs or getting injections because of their baby. Acupuncture is ideal for both the prevention and treatment of various problems associated with pregnancy.

Sciatica is a common complaint of pregnant women since the weight of the fetus puts a strain on their pelvis. I once treated a pregnant patient for sciatica, and applied direct moxibustion on SP-6 and BL-59 as part of the treatment. She had been told by her obstetrician that a cesarean section would most likely be necessary. However, with repeated acupuncture and moxibustion treatments, her condition improved and she was so pleased to be able to give birth to a healthy baby by normal delivery.

It was the obstetrician Dr. Ishino Nobuyasu who first advocated direct moxibustion on SP-6 as the treatment for easy birth. It is all the more convincing coming from an obstetrician. Recently, studies have been done in university hospitals to substantiate that acupuncture and moxibustion at SP-6 and BL-67 can correct fetal malpresentation. This is very good for our profession, and we need to inform our patients about these benefits of acupuncture.

SP-8 (chi-ki / dì jī)

(SYSTEMATIC): "Five units below the knee."

(ILLUSTRATED): "On the medial aspect of the lower leg, five units below the knee [LR-8] from the posterior border of the tibia."

LOCATION: On the medial aspect of the lower leg, one-third the distance from LR-8 to the medial malleolus, on the posterior border of the tibia (Fig. 2-73).

PALPATION: Stroke upward with the thumb from the midpoint of the tibia along its medial border. There will be a place where the finger catches. Position the thumb vertically on this point and move it back and forth along the bone to find a reaction. Since sometimes the induration is on the gastrocnemius muscle, also palpate a little posterior to the bone.

INSERTION: Use a vertical, shallow insertion.

INDICATION: Gastrointestinal diseases with acute symptoms, that is, stomach or abdominal pain, and diarrhea.

SP-9 (*in-ryō-sen / yīn líng quán*)

(SYSTEMATIC): "Below the knee on the inside, beneath the head of the tibia in the middle of the depression. Extend the leg to locate [this point]."

(ILLUSTRATED): "Stroke the posterior margin of the tibia with the leg extended. It is located in the curve of the bone where the finger comes to a stop."

LOCATION: On the posterior and inferior border of the medial condyle of the tibia (Fig. 2-73).

PALPATION: Press the upper calf with the thumb, and slide the thumb proximally along the margin of the tibia. The thumb will come to a stop where the bone starts to curve. Place the thumb or index finger vertically over this point and move it back and forth along the bone to locate a depression or tender point.

INSERTION: Use a vertical, shallow insertion. Needles can be inserted quite deeply in the points between SP-6 and SP-9, but shallow insertion is sufficient. Gently manipulate the needle at a shallow depth until you feel the arrival of qi.

INDICATION: Use for gastrointestinal diseases and problems in the knee joint when the Spleen meridian is involved. Also indicated for digestive problems when there is diarrhea or hot flashes.

SP-10 (*kek-kai / xuè hǎi*)

(SYSTEMATIC): "Above and to the inside of the knee cap, two-and-a-half units from the margin of the white flesh."

(ILLUSTRATED): "On the medial aspect of the upper leg. Two-and-a-half units above the superior medial corner of the patella. It is medial to the rectus femoris muscle, and just below the bulge of this muscle."

LOCATION: Three finger-widths above the superior medial corner of the patella (Fig. 2-73).

PALPATION: The rectus femoris muscle runs upward from the patella. When the margin of this muscle is not clear, have the patient extend the knee to make the muscles in the front bulge. Press on the margin of the muscle and move the thumb upward from the patella. Often there is a tender or indurated point where the margin of the muscle becomes indistinct. Sometimes you can find an unusually sensitive point by palpating toward the Liver meridian.

INSERTION: Use a vertical, shallow insertion with a slightly posterior and inferior direction. The needle may also be angled diagonally upward to follow the flow of the meridian.

INDICATION: Menstrual irregularity.

LR-1 *(dai-ton / dà dūn)*   ★★★

(SYSTEMATIC): "On the corner of the big toe, the width of a leek distant from [the base of] the nail, in the middle of [the point] where the three hairs reach."

(ILLUSTRATED): "One-tenth of a unit from the lateral end of the base of the big toenail."

LOCATION: On the lateral side of the big toe, 0.1 unit proximal to the corner of the toenail (Fig. 2-74).

PALPATION: Use the same technique as described for LU-11. In other words, stroke proximally along the lateral side of the toenail with the tip of the index finger until the finger comes to a small depression. Move the fingertip back and forth in this depression to locate the point.

INSERTION: Contact needling or retain the needle after superficial insertion.

INDICATION: Use for dizziness, nausea, and headaches. LR-1 is effective in cases of Liver deficiency with acute symptoms or tension or fullness in the epigastrium.

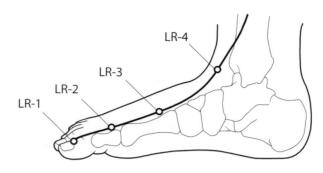

Fig. 2-74

DISCUSSION: I do not use that many points on one patient, and so the points I use fall into a certain pattern. As times goes by, this pattern of frequently used points changes. LR-1 was originally a 1-star point, which means I did not use it that often. Through the years, however, it has grown to become a favorite, a 3-star point.

Some meridian therapy practitioners say that well (wood) points should only be used for acute conditions and should not be used for chronic cases. For the symptoms I have listed, I have found that LR-1 works for chronic cases as well. Probably one reason some practitioners avoid using this point for most patients is because it can be quite painful when a needle is inserted. One good way to reduce the pain is to flick the side of the insertion tube and the needle with some force. The vibration usually gets the needle started without tapping it in from the top. Sometimes I use this technique but the patient says it still hurts. This technique works best when a metal tube is used. I use a special insertion tube where the handle of the needle protrudes only 2mm from the end of the tube prior to insertion. Disposable needles with plastic tubes do not work as well, but with practice, the pain of insertion can be minimized.

Once, a 58-year-old man from another prefecture came to my clinic for treatment. He had a headache over his entire head that had lasted for over five months. He was examined by a neurologist but was told that there was nothing wrong. He also had insomnia, numbness in his fingertips, and some lower back pain. His diastolic blood pressure was a little high at 90mmHg. I wanted this patient to get relief soon, especially because he came from far away and could not be treated often. I thought that perhaps he could receive home moxibustion treatments on his back points, but I learned he had lost his wife and there was no one who could give him moxibustion treatments at home. Under these circumstances, I marked LR-1 and LR-3 on both feet and told him to apply direct moxibustion on himself every day.

His condition was greatly improved after the second treatment. Direct moxibustion on LR-1 can be quite painful, but this patient did not complain. I guess the pain is not so bad when you are already in pain.

LR-2 (*kō-kan / xíng jiān*)

(*SYSTEMATIC*): "Between the big toes, in the middle of the depression with the pulsation."

(*ILLUSTRATED*): "[It is on] the web between the first and second toes, on the margin of the red and white flesh."

LOCATION: Between the first and second toes, anterior to the metatarsophalangeal joints (Fig. 2-74).

PALPATION: Place the thumb between the first and second toes distal to the joint. Press toward the big toe and move over the webbing toward the metatarsophalangeal joint. Palpate the joint carefully to find a tender point. It is helpful to move the fingertip slightly back and forth along the bone as you press. As previously discussed under LI-2, depending on which classical source one is using, LR-2 can be either distal or proximal to the "main joint." Either location is good so long as there is a clear reaction.

INSERTION: Use a diagonal, shallow insertion with the needle aimed proximally and medially.

INDICATION: LR-2 is a dispersion point for Liver excess. It is useful for headaches and nausea related to a Liver imbalance.

DISCUSSION: When the Liver pulse (left middle position) is very strong while the Lung and Spleen pulses (right distal and middle positions) are weak, tonifying the Lung and Spleen meridians alone is not sufficient to reduce the Liver excess. Also, it does not alleviate attendant symptoms such as headache, lower back pain, and tension in the abdomen. In such cases, needling LR-2 improves the pulse along with the symptoms.

LR-3 (*tai-shō / tài chōng*)

(*SYSTEMATIC*): "Two units behind the main joint of the big toe."

(*ILLUSTRATED*): "When the space between the first and second toes is pressed from LR-2, [and the finger is moved] proximally between the bones, there is a place where the finger comes to a stop at the head of the metatarsal where it bulges up. Furthermore, the pulsation of the anterior tibial artery can be felt. Locate the point here."

LOCATION: In the depression distal to the point where the first and second metatarsals meet (Fig. 2-74).

PALPATION: Stroking proximally with the middle finger between the first and second toes, the finger comes to a stop where the metatarsals join. Use the tip of the thumb to press above and below this point. Move the thumb back and forth as you press in toward the first metatarsal, as if you are trying to get under the bone. In other words, you should look for reactions, not between the metatarsals, but along the first metatarsal.

INSERTION: Use a diagonal, shallow insertion with the needle aimed either proximally or distally toward the big toe. This point must be needled carefully or else there can be a strong sensation.

INDICATION: Used both for tonification and dispersion in cases of Liver imbalance. LR-3 is especially useful in cases of Liver deficiency with loss of appetite. Also, because it is the source point of the Liver meridian, I prescribe it for home moxibustion treatments.

LR-4 (*chū-hō / zhōng fēng*)

(*VITAL AXIS*): "One-and-a-half units in front of the medial malleolus in the middle of the depression. Find [this point] by moving the foot back and forth."

(*ILLUSTRATED*): "Half a unit in front of the medial malleolus, in the depression. There are three big tendons on the front of the foot. From medial to lateral, they are the tendons of the tibialis anterior, extensor hallucis longus, and extensor digitorum longus muscles. LR-4 is located on the medial border of the tendon of the tibialis anterior. This is half way between SP-5 and ST-41."

(*ESSENTIAL POINTS*): "It is where the finger comes to a stop when sliding it along the medial border of the tendon of the tibialis anterior. Move the foot to locate."

LOCATION: 1.5 units anterior to the medial malleolus on the medial border of the tendon of the tibialis anterior (Fig. 2-74).

PALPATION: The thumb or index finger are best for palpating LR-4. Place a finger in the depression between the navicular bone and the medial malleolus (SP-5), and slide the finger forward to find the tendon of the tibialis anterior. Position the finger vertically to palpate along the tendon.

As implied in *Location of Essential Points,* the reaction for LR-4 is sometimes quite a bit distal along the tendon. This is especially the case for indurations. However, sensitivity to pinching is usually found at the standard location. LR-4 is one of the distal points that can be very painful when pinched.

INSERTION: Use a vertical, shallow insertion.

INDICATION: Coughing, wheezing, and fevers in cases of Liver deficiency.

DISCUSSION: LR-4 is easier to locate and needle than LR-8. Sometimes, when I am in a hurry and patients are wearing pants that do not roll up easily, I use LR-3 or LR-4, instead of LR-8, to tonify the Liver meridian.

According to one of my senior students, Shibahara Toshi-ichi, he treated a middle-aged female patient who came in with a cold and a high fever. His diagnosis was Liver deficiency, and he found a marked response on LR-4 on one side, so he applied direct moxibustion. The patient felt the heat at first, but then quickly stopped feeling it. After about 60 cones, the heat sensation returned so he stopped applying moxa. Just this moxibustion treatment reduced the patient's fever and relieved her symptoms.

LR-5 (*rei-kō / lǐ gōu*)

(WANG, 1027): "In the depression."

(SYSTEMATIC): "The connecting point of the *jue yin* of the leg, it is five units above the medial malleolus."

(ILLUSTRATED): "Medial aspect of calf, five units above the medial malleolus on the medial surface of the tibia. It is 0.2 to 0.3 unit anterior to the [posterior] margin of the bone, on the surface of the bone where there is no muscle."

LOCATION: One-third the distance from the medial malleolus to the knee, in the depression on the medial surface of the tibia (Fig. 2-75).

PALPATION: Work your way up the surface of the tibia from about one-third of the

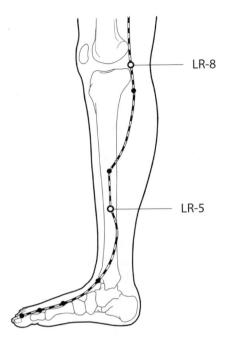

Fig. 2-75

way up, pressing with the base of your thumb. There will be a depression with marked tenderness. It is in the center of the medial surface of the tibia.

INSERTION: Use a vertical, shallow insertion.

INDICATION: LR-5 is useful as the connecting point of the Liver meridian. In other words, it is used when there is an imbalance in the Liver meridian and a reaction is palpated. It is also a useful point for treating the Liver meridian with direct moxibustion.

LR-8 (*kyoku-sen* / *qǔ quán*)   ★★★

(*SYSTEMATIC*): "Below the medial condyle of the knee, on the big muscle, below the little muscle, in the middle of the depression. Find [this point] by flexing the knee."

(ILLUSTRATED): "In the depression on the medial aspect of the knee. It is at the end of the crease when the knee is [fully] flexed. It is between the sartorius and gracilis muscles."

LOCATION: In the depression on the medial aspect of the knee (Fig. 2-75).

PALPATION: A depression can be found when stroking the medial aspect of the knee with the pad of a finger. Place the fingertip in the most depressed point and move it back and forth slightly in a vertical direction, up and down. There will be tenderness or an induration. Locate the point over the reaction. This might be called an 'excess point within a deficient area'.

INSERTION: Use a diagonal, shallow insertion with the needle pointed proximally. The needle may be retained.

INDICATION: LR-8 is the principal tonification point for Liver deficiency. The symptomatic applications of this point are many and include nausea, dizziness, pain in the lower abdomen, headache, lower back pain, and knee pain.

DISCUSSION: Although LR-8 is effective for dizziness, on a rare occasion it can cause dizziness. I once retained a needle shallowly in LR-8 on a patient, which I do all the time, and he started feeling dizzy. I often retain needles shallowly in other tonification points such as KI-7, SP-3, LU-9, PC-7, KI-10, and LU-5, but I have no experience of these points causing such symptoms as dizziness in a patient. Aside from the issue of a misdiagnosis, it is perplexing that retaining a needle in LR-8 could actually cause dizziness. I have never had a case where simple insertion in LR-8 caused dizziness. In the *Journal of the Japan Meridian Therapy Association*, Ikeda Masakazu has argued that retaining a needle in tonification points for root treatment is a questionable practice. He suggests that it might cause a leakage or loss of qi.

The approach of retaining many shallowly inserted needles is said to have been developed by Okabe Sodo, one of the founders of meridian therapy. Due to his influence, in my practice I tend to retain needles more often than simply inserting them. Retaining the needle can work either way, however, so you have to be careful about the opposite effect. You need to be especially careful about retaining needles in distal points of the Lung and Liver meridians, which, in my experience, are more sensitive and require more care than other points. Also, it is a problem if your repertoire is limited to retaining needles. One must master different techniques, and one must especially learn to feel the arrival of qi at the point.

LR-8 can be a difficult point to needle on patients who are sensitive or have thin skin. It is especially hard to get the needle started without pain. To needle LR-8, some practitioners have the patient externally rotate the hip, and flex the knee slightly, and support the leg with a small pillow. This makes it easier to get the needle started and to retain the needle. It is crucial that one become proficient at needling the tonification points. The more you use them, the better you become at needling them. This does not necessarily mean that you will have an easy time or get the intended results every time. As with any other art, each time you do it, you reach a higher level and greater possibilities appear.

GB-29 (*kyo-ryō / jū liáo*)

(SYSTEMATIC): "Eight-and-three-tenths units below LR-13, above the protruding bone, in the middle of the depression."

(ILLUSTRATED): "Posterior to the origin of the sartorius muscle at the anterior superior iliac spine. In the depression at the origin of the tensor fascia latae. Apply pressure and locate [this point] where there is pain."

LOCATION: Three finger-widths medial and inferior to the anterior superior iliac spine (Fig. 2-76).

PALPATION: The inguinal ligament runs in a medial and inferior direction from the anterior superior iliac spine. Locate the tightest point on the lateral portion of this ligament.

INSERTION: Use a vertical, shallow insertion in the hardest point.

INDICATION: Use for hip joint problems. I also check GB-29 for a reaction when the Iliac point is tender or indurated. When there is a strong reaction, I treat both GB-29 and the Iliac point.

KI-1 (*yū-sen / yǒng quán*)

(SYSTEMATIC): "On the sole of the foot, in the depression. Flex the foot and toes to curl them up; [the point] is in the bowl-like depression."

(ILLUSTRATED): "It is in the depression in the sole created by flexing the five toes.

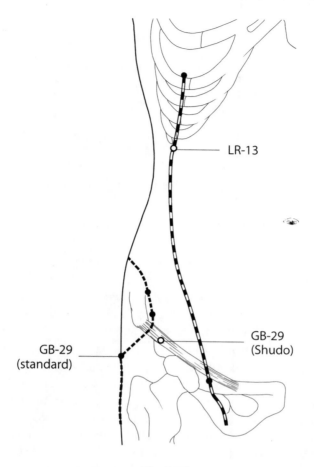

LR-13

GB-29
(Shudo)

GB-29
(standard)

Fig. 2-76

It is between the bones of the second and third metatarsals and is slightly medial to the center of the transverse crease."

LOCATION: On the anterior aspect of the sole of the foot, in the deepest part of the depression when the toes are fully flexed (Fig. 2-77).

PALPATION: When all the toes are flexed, a crease or depression forms in the sole. You can bend the toes or have the patient flex the toes. Press the tip of your thumb in the middle of this depression and often you will find a tender point or an induration. The reaction often appears anterior to the standard location. Be sure to palpate on, as well as between, the metatarsals.

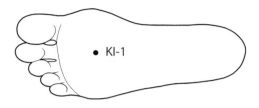

Fig. 2-77

INSERTION: Use a vertical, superficial insertion. Insert the needle swiftly, or else it can be painful. Do not retain the needle.

INDICATION: For raising energy, invigorating, and reviving consciousness. Use direct moxibustion to resuscitate.

DISCUSSION: This incident took place years ago while I was studying with my teacher, Master Miura. He had a daughter who was a high school student at the time. She had a convulsion in the middle of the night and lost consciousness. I am not sure what the cause was, but from what I could gather, it must have been epilepsy. My teacher, being a very emotional man, unlike his usual self, became all flustered and was at a loss for what to do. There was a woman relative who was staying with him at the time, and she asked him why he did not do moxibustion on KI-1. She had seen my teacher do this on other patients. My teacher came to himself and started applying moxibustion on KI-1, as suggested, and his daughter regained consciousness in a short while. It is surprising how this man who was so calm and efficient when treating me when I was critically ill with anemia from chronic diarrhea, became so flustered when it came to treating his own daughter. From this I concluded that the practice of having someone else treat the family members of physicians and therapists makes sense.

Moxibustion on KI-1 is also an effective way for reducing blood pressure in cases of hypertension and arteriosclerosis. Some authors caution against doing moxibustion on the top of the head and the occipital area in cases of hypertension. I strongly agree. I used to treat many patients who had strokes, and I wondered about the use of direct moxibustion in such cases.

Re-reading Honma's *The Illustrated Manual to Practical Acupuncture and Moxibustion Points,* I found a passage which addresses this issue directly:

> Direct moxibustion is generally very effective for those who tend toward hot flashes, high blood pressure, and hardening of the arteries. In some cases, however, this treatment can increase the rebellious flow of qi, and tinnitus or tension in the neck

and shoulders gets worse. It seems that moxibustion on GV-20 is not so good for those who have a reddish or puffy face, strong tinnitus, blurred vision, or are mentally unclear. I have had a bad experience of causing retinal bleeding by applying direct moxibustion on GV-20 at the request of a patient who had high blood pressure. I will never forget how I regretted forgetting that in cases like this, acupuncture is used to disperse the cranial area and moxibustion is applied on points on the foot like KI-1.

This is so true. Just because there are symptoms in a certain place does not mean that area should be treated. One must know how to treat distal points on the arms and legs. Sometimes the direct method works for you, and sometimes it works against you.

KI-2 (*nen-koku / rán gǔ*)   ★★

(*SYSTEMATIC*): "In front of the medial malleolus, under the navicular bone, in the middle of the depression."

(*ILLUSTRATED*): "The navicular bone is the prominent bone anterior and inferior to the medial malleolus. [This point] is under its lower margin, and it is located in the depression between [this bone] and the medial cuneiform bone. It is painful when pressed."

LOCATION: In the depression under the navicular bone (Fig. 2-78).

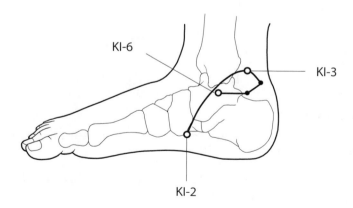

Fig. 2-78

PALPATION: There is a protruding bone anterior and inferior to KI-6, that is, the navicular bone, and underneath it there is a depression. Find the point that is most depressed by pressing with a fingertip. The point is often tender.

INSERTION: Use a vertical, superficial insertion.

INDICATION: This point is useful for tinnitus, hot feet, and parotitis (also called parotiditis). Direct moxibustion on KI-2 is effective for removing dampness in ear diseases.

DISCUSSION: Direct moxibustion on KI-2 works wonders for suppurations and other excretions from the ear, as well as fluid in the ear from otitis media. My patients who have been going to ear-nose-throat (ENT) specialists for months surprise their doctors because their infected ear dries up so quickly as a result of moxibustion. For some reason, acupuncture at KI-2 does not have such a dramatic effect.

Sometimes it happens that a bad case of *katakori* (neck and shoulder stiffness), which almost makes a person sick, is actually caused by an accumulation of fluids in the ear, especially in elderly women. If you suspect this, have the patient see a specialist and get the problem treated. Then apply direct moxibustion on KI-2 to consolidate the effect.

Multiple cones of direct moxibustion on KI-2 is effective for parotitis, which causes swelling under the ears. In this case, often no pain is felt when moxibustion is applied to KI-2. It is amazing, but applying more cones until the heat is felt clears up the heat, swelling, and pain in the jaw.

KI-3 (*tai-kei / tài xī*)

(SYSTEMATIC): "Behind the medial malleolus, above the calcaneus, in the depression with the pulsation."

(ILLUSTRATED): "Half a unit posterior to the margin of the medial malleolus, where there is a pulsation."

LOCATION: Posterior to the medial malleolus where the pulsation of the posterior tibial artery is strongest (Fig. 2-78).

PALPATION: First, find the pulsation with your fingertip. If the pulsation is clear, locate the point where the pulsation is strongest. When the pulsation is weak or hard to feel, look for a tender or indurated point. This area is usually so depressed, however, that it is hard to find tenderness and induration. So I like to dorsiflex the ankle with one hand and use the tip of the thumb or the middle finger of the other hand to palpate with a small circular motion. When locating the point for root treatment, it is sufficient to stroke lightly with a fingertip to find the most depressed point.

INSERTION: Use a vertical, shallow insertion. The needle may move slightly with the pulsation. Deep needling will reach the nerve to produce a radiating sensation in the sole of the foot. One must be careful because sensitive patients dislike such strong sensations and it serves to disperse qi.

INDICATION: KI-3 is the source point of the Kidney meridian so it is often used to treat Kidney deficiency. If asked about a specific application for this point, I would say cases of Kidney deficiency with digestive problems, such as a lack of appetite. This is because KI-3 is the earth point of the Kidney meridian. The earth points, which are also the source points on the yin meridians, serve to tonify the Spleen and Stomach in addition to having other effects. KI-3 is often used along with KI-6 for moxibustion treatments. The point is also handy for the self-treatment of Kidney deficiency.

DISCUSSION: Some texts say that the abnormalities in the yin organs are reflected in the source points:

> Where there is disease in the five yin organs, the reaction is found in the twelve source [points] ... Injury to the five yin organs becomes known by having clear knowledge of these source [points] and looking for their reaction. When there is disease in the five yin organs, the twelve source [points] should be treated straight-away. (*Vital Axis*, Chapter 1)

In other words, palpating reactions at the source points enables us to determine the presence or absence of disease in the five yin organs. When there is a reaction, that source point can be used to treat the disease. This is the classical concept of source points, and it has clinical validity.

In the classics, one often finds the term '*shao yin* vessel' in reference to the Kidney meridian. This term is used repeatedly in the *Pulse Classic* (Wang Shu-He, 280). Kosoto Yo, a prominent Japanese classical scholar, points out, however, that this term is borrowed from earlier classics like *Discussion of Cold-Induced Disorders* and *Essentials from the Golden Cabinet* (Kosoto, 1981). Both of these texts were originally written by Zhang Zhong-Jing in the early third century. "The *shao yin* vessel is tight and submerged. Tight indicates pain, and submerged indicates damp-ness. Therefore, urination is difficult." (Zhang, c. 220). Thus, when the *shao yin* ves-sel is submerged and tight, one can surmise that there is pain and difficulty with urination. "[This is] primarily a diagnostic method for determining the urological and reproductive functions related to the function of the Kidney." (Maruyama, 1977)

In other words, the pulsation at KI-3, or the *shao yin* pulse, was palpated to diagnose the condition of the Kidneys and Bladder as well as the Kidney and Bladder meridians. This method is seldom used now since six-position pulse diag-nosis was developed. Recently, however, some herbalists and meridian therapy practitioners have been experimenting with the method. This endeavor is very interesting, especially because of the aging of the population and the connection between the Kidney, aging, and the bones and marrow.

KI-6 (*shō-kai / zhào hǎi*)   ★

(*SYSTEMATIC*): "One unit below the medial malleolus."

(*ILLUSTRATED*): "Approximately one finger-width below the medial malleolus, there is a groove between the ligament and tendon. Locate [KI-6] in this depres-sion. There is pain with strong pressure."

LOCATION: One unit below the medial malleolus (Fig. 2-78).

PALPATION: Press the tip of the thumb into a point one or two finger-widths below the high point of the medial malleolus. The point is in the center of the hardest spot over the bone.

INSERTION: Use a vertical, superficial insertion.

INDICATION: Throat pain.

KI-7 (*fuku-ryū / fù liū*)   ★★★

(*SYSTEMATIC*): "Two units above the medial malleolus in the middle of the depression."

(*ILLUSTRATED*): "Two units above the upper margin of the medial malleolus on the anterior border of the Achilles tendon."

LOCATION: Two units above the medial malleolus on the anterior border of the Achilles tendon (Fig. 2-79).

PALPATION: Often a depression can be found when stroking with a fingertip the anterior border of the Achilles tendon in a proximal direction. KI-7 is located in the most depressed area above KI-3 along the Achilles tendon. If there is no depression, palpate toward the tibia from two units above the medial malleolus and locate the most tender point.

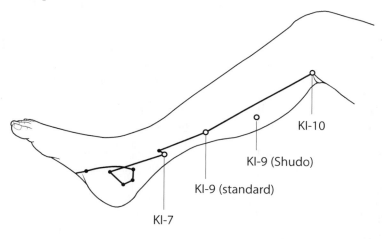

Fig. 2-79

INSERTION: Use a diagonal insertion with the needle pointed proximally.

INDICATION: KI-7 is the principal tonification point for Kidney deficiency. It is therefore effective for symptoms such as distention in the lower abdomen, tendency to become fatigued, lack of libido, loss of balance, tinnitus, and tendency to become chilled.

DISCUSSION: There are no indications given for KI-7 in Shiroda's *Basic Study of Acupuncture and Moxibustion Therapy,* the bible of Sawada-style acupuncture. Since we practiced this style, my teacher and I never used KI-7. I had an extremely hard induration at KI-7 on my left ankle. My teacher told me that something as hard as this was not in the same category as indurations and tender points, both of which are the targets of treatment in the Sawada style. Nevertheless, it was clearly related to the Kidney meridian, considering my history of peritonitis with hemoptysis, hemorrhoids, and difficulty standing for a long time.

In *Japanese Classical Acupuncture: Introduction to Meridian Therapy* I told the story of how needling KI-7 had a remarkable effect in relieving distention in my lower abdomen. This was all the more remarkable since I had bypassed this point for so long. I realized that changing your perspective can sometimes open up a whole new dimension. This is true not only of which points we choose to use, but also of the approach we use. It is a shame to insist that there is only one way to do something, and never go beyond that.

KI-9 (*chiku-bin / zhú bīn*)

(*SYSTEMATIC*): "Above the medial malleolus, in between the muscle of the calf."

(*ILLUSTRATED*): "Five units above the medial malleolus, on the anterior border of the Achilles tendon in the flexor hallucis longus muscle."

LOCATION: On the medial aspect of the calf, one-third of the way from the medial crease of the knee to the medial malleolus, in the belly of the gastrocnemius muscle (Fig. 2-79).

PALPATION: Find the tightest point on the medial aspect of the gastrocnemius muscle. Probe for this point with the tip of your thumb or middle finger using a circular motion.

INSERTION: Use a vertical, superficial insertion.

INDICATION: KI-9 is useful for imbalances in the Kidney meridian, especially when there are acute symptoms such as palpitations, heart pain, or chest pain. Perhaps this effect comes from KI-9 being the cleft point of the Yin Heel vessel (*in kyō myaku/yīn qiāo mài*). I retain an intradermal needle in KI-9 for the prevention of motion sickness.

DISCUSSION: KI-9 is often sensitive to pinching, and this can be used as an aid in diagnosis as well as for treatment. The location of this point varies a great deal, moving up or down as well as forward or backward. It should be regarded as an area instead of a point. I used to use this KI-9 area for almost every case of Kidney or Liver meridian imbalance when there was a reaction, but these days I tend to use KI-7 or KI-10 instead. This change is due to my experience that good results can be obtained without the use of many points on the same meridian. Or maybe I am getting lazy in my old age.

An intradermal needle retained in the most reactive point in the KI-9 area works wonders for motion sickness. I have a colleague who claims that an intradermal needle in SP-6 is better, but I tend to use KI-9. Using both points would cover all the bases, but I think that retaining a needle in the most indurated and tender point on just one side is sufficient.

The important thing is the location. Most textbooks place KI-9 one-third or one-quarter of the way from the medial malleolus to the medial crease of the knee. For preventing motion sickness, however, I have found that one-third of the way down from the knee works better. In my experience among the adults I have treated, other than one patient who almost became sick and another who became sick the day after treatment, no one had motion sickness. It does not work as well with elementary school children. About ten percent of them seem to get motion sickness anyway. Therefore, I cannot guarantee this treatment as being one-hundred percent effective. Nevertheless, it is a very simple and effective measure for preventing motion sickness.

KI-10 (*in-koku / yīn gǔ*)   ★★★

(*SYSTEMATIC*): "Below the knee, behind the medial condyle, under the big tendon, and above the little tendon. When [this point is] pressed, it can be felt in the hand. Locate with the knee flexed."

(*ILLUSTRATED*): "When the tendons medial and posterior to the knee are stroked with the fingers with the knee flexed at a 90° angle, there is [a] thick tendon that is most posterior and a thinner tendon just lateral to that and a finger can be put in between them. The point is medial to BL-40, in this space between the tendons."

(*ESSENTIAL POINTS*): "On the medial aspect of the popliteal fossa. Flex the knee a little [to locate it] or [have the patient] lie supine. [It is] between the tendons of the semitendinosus and gastrocnemius muscles."

LOCATION: On the medial aspect of the popliteal fossa between the tendons of the semitendinosus and semimembranosus muscles. Locate this point with the knee slightly flexed (Fig. 2-79).

PALPATION: Two tendons can be palpated on the medial side of the popliteal fossa when the knee is bent a little and the leg is relaxed. KI-10 is located between these two tendons. When the knee is extended, a slight depression appears medial to LR-8.

Stroke lightly with a fingertip to locate this depression.

INSERTION: KI-10 is easier to locate and needle with the knee slightly flexed. Insert diagonally with the tip pointed proximally. Superficial and shallow insertions both seem to work on this point, but I generally insert less than 5mm.

INDICATION: Tonification point for Kidney and Liver deficiency patterns.

DISCUSSION: KI-10 is the water point of the water phase meridian. Therefore, the point manifests the water aspect of the Kidney. In Chapter 23 of *Vital Axis* it is noted that "water pertains to the Kidney." This means that the Kidney is involved with everything related to water or fluids. When you think about the fact that the body is composed mostly of water, it makes sense that the Kidney meridian covers many different aspects of our bodily functions. There are many varieties of body fluids including tears, nasal discharge, sputum, urine, edema, and lymph. KI-10 should come to mind as a useful point when there is a problem with any one of these.

ST-41 (kai-kei / jĭe xī)

(VITAL AXIS): "One-and-a-half units above ST-42 in the middle of the depression."

(ILLUSTRATED): "In the center of the anterior aspect of the ankle joint. [It is] located in the small depression when the foot is in slight plantar flexion."

LOCATION: Between the tendons on the anterior aspect of the ankle. From a medial to lateral direction, there are the tendons of the tibialis anterior, extensor hallucis longus, and extensor digitorum longus muscles. ST-41 is located over the tendon of the extensor hallucis longus (Fig. 2-80).

PALPATION: Palpate the tendons on the front of the ankle and find the depression between the tendons of the tibialis anterior and extensor digitorum longus muscles.

INSERTION: Use a vertical, shallow insertion.

INDICATION: ST-41 is the fire point of the Stomach meridian and is therefore useful for tonification when the Stomach meridian is deficient. Agario Mitsuru, one of the practitioners in my local study group, likes to pinch the sternocleidomastoid

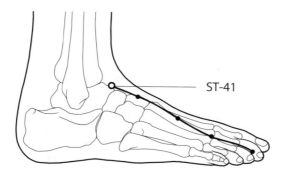

Fig. 2-80

muscle before his treatments to see if there is any tenderness, which he attributes to deficiency of the Stomach meridian. If there is a great deal of tenderness, he retains a needle in ST-41 on the same side. He says that the tenderness usually disappears by the end of the treatment.

ST-40   (*hō-ryū / fēng lóng*)

(*SYSTEMATIC*): "Eight units above the lateral malleolus, on the lateral margin of the tibia, in the middle of the depression."

(*ILLUSTRATED*): "On the lateral side of the anterior aspect of the lower leg, eight units above the lateral malleolus. It is one unit lateral to ST-38. Locate close to the groove in the muscle."

LOCATION: On the lower leg, halfway between the bottom of the patella and the lateral malleolus, on the lateral margin of the tibialis anterior muscle (Fig. 2-81).

PALPATION: Stroke downward with four fingers from ST-36 to ST-39, and then palpate the lateral margin of the tibialis anterior muscle. Press down into the groove between the muscles to find the most indurated point.

INSERTION: Use a vertical, superficial insertion.

INDICATION: Use when there is an imbalance in the Stomach meridian. I often use ST-40 to disperse Stomach meridian excess.

201

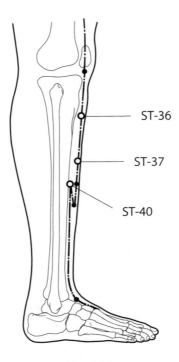

ST-36

ST-37

ST-40

Fig. 2-81

ST-37 (*jō-ko-kyo / shàng jù xū*)   ★

(SYSTEMATIC): "Three units below ST-36."

(ILLUSTRATED): "Three units below ST-36 in the tibialis anterior muscle."

LOCATION: Approximately three finger-widths below ST-36 in the tibialis anterior muscle (Fig. 2-81).

PALPATION: Hook the thumb and press in the muscle successively downward from ST-36. Find the tightest point about three units below ST-36.

INSERTION: Use a vertical or diagonal, superficial insertion with the needle pointing proximally.

INDICATION: Direct moxibustion is most effective for knee pain when there is edema.

DISCUSSION: Locating and treating reactive points around the knee is generally sufficient to treat arthritic knee pain. When there is edema, however, imbalances in the meridians must be treated; otherwise, the edema is usually not resolved. The Liver meridian is often deficient when there are arthritic knee conditions, while edema of the knees is generally associated with a deficiency in the Kidney or Spleen meridian. Of the yang meridians, the Stomach meridian is most often involved and should be treated. Among the points of the Stomach meridian, reactive points between ST-37 and ST-39 are most useful, and direct moxibustion on these points sometimes quickly resolves the edema. I use these points on the Stomach meridian to reduce swelling in the knee regardless of the chief complaint or the meridian imbalance.

I have a female patient who was over 70-years old when she first came for treatment with chronic swelling in her knees. She was having fluid removed every week at a local hospital, but the swelling would not go away. She was on her way to another acupuncture clinic when the taxi driver told her about mine. It took many treatments to reduce the swelling in her knees, but I have been seeing her for more than a dozen years and she is now well into her eighties. She attributes her longevity to regular acupuncture treatments. But there is a downside to this. She has outlived her husband and only son, and it is not easy living alone. Ironically, her visits to my clinic have now become more important to her than ever.

ST-36 (*ashi-san-li / zú sān lǐ*)

(BASIC QUESTIONS): "When [this point is] pressed very hard, the pulsation on the top of the foot [ST-41] ceases."

(SYSTEMATIC): "Three units below the knee, on the lateral margin of the tibia."

(ESSENTIAL POINTS): "Lateral to the tibial tuberosity. Next to the point where the finger comes to a stop when stroking up the anterior surface of the tibia. In the tibialis anterior muscle, three units below the eye of the knee [M-LE-16]."

LOCATION: Two finger-widths lateral to the tuberosity of the tibia, in the tibialis anterior muscle (Fig. 2-81).

PALPATION: Locate this point with the knee extended. Stroke upward on the anterior and medial margin of the tibia to find the tuberosity of the tibia. The origin of the tibialis anterior muscle is two finger-widths lateral to this. Press this area with the tip of the thumb as you work it up and down or across the muscle to locate the tightest point.

INSERTION: Use a vertical or diagonal insertion with the tip pointing superiorly. Generally, shallow insertion is sufficient. Be careful not to cause a strong sensation by inserting deeper into the tibialis anterior muscle.

INDICATION: ST-36 is used to tonify the Spleen and Stomach. It is effective for digestive problems, insomnia, depression, and knee problems with edema.

DISCUSSION: In Honma's *The Illustrated Manual to Practical Acupuncture and Moxibustion Points,* ST-36 is located at the midpoint between the tibial tuberosity and the head of the fibula. In Shiroda's *Basic Study of Acupuncture and Moxibustion Therapy,* ST-36 is "at the center point of the line connecting the point one unit below the head of the fibula and the inferior margin of the tuberosity of the tibia." ST-36 is supposed to be in the middle of the tibialis anterior muscle, but these locations place ST-36 on the lateral margin of the muscle. In my experience, the tightest points on the tibialis anterior are to be found right up close to the tibia.

In *Basic Questions* it is noted that the location of ST-36 can be determined by pressing hard on the point to stop the pulsation at the dorsalis pedis artery. Other texts also suggest this method, but if occlusion of the artery is all that is required, ST-37, ST-38, or ST-39 serve just as well.

M-LE-16 *(shitsu-gan / xī yǎn; (ST-35) toku-bi / dú bí)*   ★★

(SUN, 700): "Below the patella in the depression on either side. In the middle of the bowl-like depression."

(ILLUSTRATED): "Below the patella in the depression on either side of the patellar tendon."

LOCATION: In the depressions medial and lateral to the patellar tendon (Fig. 2-82).

PALPATION: Locate this point with the leg extended. The location inside the depressions is simple enough, but I have a special technique for finding the reactive point. For the left knee, I stand on the left side of the patient and use the palmar aspect of my right distal thumb joint to palpate the depression medial to the patellar tendon. A reaction (induration or tender point) is found by pressing and moving the thumb joint back and forth or up and down. I use the distal thumb joint of my left hand to palpate the depression lateral to the patellar tendon. For the right

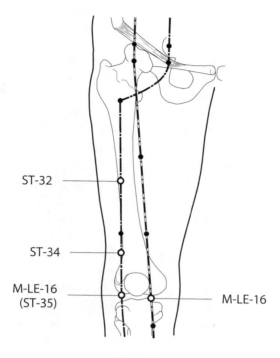

ST-32

ST-34

M-LE-16
(ST-35)

M-LE-16

Fig. 2-82

knee, I stand on the right side of the patient and use the opposite thumb joints from those described above.

INSERTION: Use a vertical insertion with the leg extended; a shallow insertion is best.

INDICATION: Knee pain and arthritis.

DISCUSSION: It is said that the process of degeneration or aging in our body begins around the age of twenty-five. In the blood vessels, stenosis (narrowing) of the vertebral artery comes first, and among the joints, the knee is the first to show signs of degeneration. Indurations and tenderness around the joint are signs of degeneration, and in fact you can detect some degeneration in most patients when you palpate around the knee joint, as explained above. Often the patient has no pain or problem in the knee, but there are small lumps or 'gummy' points that feel different from the surrounding area. It may be many years before the patient has any knee pain, but it is too late by the time they notice it, possibly receiving a diagnosis of osteoarthritis. The asymptomatic state with reactive points but no pain can be compared to an inactive volcano, which may become active at any time.

A reactive point can often be located in the depression lateral to the patellar tendon by palpating with the distal thumb joint. When it comes to the depression medial to the patellar tendon, however, the reaction rarely appears in the depression. I find that the reaction is usually more medial and superior to the depression on the medial side of the tendon. When the point is located precisely, the needle does not have to be inserted very deeply at all. Sometimes just rotating the needle close to the surface produces a pleasant needle sensation. This is enough.

A common way to treat knee pain in Japan is to apply direct moxibustion at the medial and lateral *shitsu-gan* points and at ST-34 and SP-10. The effect is limited, however, when the points are not reactive. When there is degeneration in the knee joint, it is of little use to treat points around the knee unless you pinpoint the reactive points. Repeated moxibustion treatments on standard points will not bring the desired results. The important thing, after all, is to locate one or two points that are really tender. I used to treat knee problems by doing deep insertions in both the medial and lateral *shitsu-gan* points with the knee flexed. But this direct approach now seems like the long way around. Knee problems increase as patients age, and direct moxibustion that can be done at home by the patient is the most simple and effective approach. The more I treat chronic knee problems, the more I feel that moxibustion is really the root treatment. Moxibustion is also useful for facilitating healing after knee surgery.

Acute arthritis in the knee, however, is quite another matter. Every point you press around the knee is likely to be painful. I recently treated a 42-year-old woman with arthritis in the knee. She experienced some pain in her right knee the evening before she came in for treatment. During that night, the knee pain became so bad that even her clothes touching the knee became unbearable. She could barely walk and had difficulty coming to my clinic. Her right knee was red, swollen, and warm all around the patella, and tender all over. Her pulse was floating and slow, and the Kidney position was deficient while the Bladder, Gallbladder, and Stomach positions were excessive. On her abdomen there was tenderness at KI-16 on the left.

In acute cases like this, local treatment must be kept to a minimum. I retained needles in both KI-7 and then successively needled KI-10, ST-40, BL-40, BL-23, and BL-25 without retaining. I did some contact needling around the affected area, and then placed an intradermal needle in M-LE-16 just below the patella. When the patient came in two days later for another treatment, the inflammation and tenderness were greatly reduced, and she was able to walk without difficulty. Her symptoms resolved completely after the second treatment. One must be careful in treating acute cases like this because overtreatment can exacerbate the problem.

ST-34 (*ryō-kyū / liáng qīu*)

(SUN, 700): "Two units above the knee."

(ILLUSTRATED): "On the anterior aspect of the thigh, two units above the lateral superior corner of the patella. There is a small depression in the vastus lateralis muscle. It is painful when pressed."

LOCATION: Approximately three finger-widths above the lateral superior corner of the patella. It is lateral to the tendon of the rectus femoris (Fig. 2-82).

PALPATION: Press and move the finger back and forth across the muscle as you work your way upward from the lateral superior corner of the patella. There will be a tender point in a groove between the muscles two or three finger-widths above the patella. Also, if the tender point is not obvious, try moving the finger back and forth along the muscle.

INSERTION: Use a vertical, superficial insertion. Retaining an intradermal needle is also effective.

INDICATION: Knee pain.

DISCUSSION: Back when I used to do house calls, I remember placing an intradermal needle in ST-34 for a patient who had edema and spontaneous pain in the knee. When I went to treat the patient again, he told me that a pricking sensation had persisted where I had placed the intradermal needle. I must have accidentally placed the needle diagonally instead of horizontally. In any case, the edema was reduced considerably the next day, and so the patient was very impressed. The irritation caused by the intradermal needle was unintentional, but it must have worked in my favor.

ST-32 (*fuku-to / fú tù*)

(VITAL AXIS): "Six units above the knee, between the bulging muscles."

(ILLUSTRATED): "Palpate the lateral border of the rectus femoris muscle and locate [this point] six units above the lateral superior corner of the patella."

LOCATION: In the center of the anterolateral aspect of the thigh, in line with the lateral superior corner of the patella (Fig. 2-82).

PALPATION: There is a point on the anterolateral aspect of the thigh about midway between the knee and the anterior superior illiac spine where the skin is especially thick when pinched. The patient feels a sharp or pricking sensation when pinched here. This point can also be found by lightly striking the middle of the anterolateral thigh.

INSERTION: Use a vertical, shallow insertion. However, sometimes the insertion has to be deep to reach the induration.

INDICATION: Neuralgia of the femoral cutaneous nerve .

DISCUSSION: I have another story about Master Miura, my teacher. As the cleft point of the Stomach meridian, ST-34 is commonly used for acute stomach pain. Master Miura used to say that ST-32 worked better, and he often needled ST-32 on himself. It seems he acquired this habit in the early years of his practice. When his teacher, the famous meridian therapy practitioner Yanagiya Sorei, came to visit his clinic, I asked Yanagiya about my teacher's preference for ST-32. Yanagiya responded in a noncommital way, "If that's what he thinks, that's fine." He looked a little perplexed, however, and did not seem particularly pleased about it. That was his way. Yanagiya never compelled his students to follow his ideas and instead allowed them to go their own ways. Due to Yanagiya's hands-off approach, and the fact that Master Miura was older and more experienced in life as a lawyer, made their relationship ambivalent. So my teacher did not absorb much of Yanagiya's knowledge and philosophy, and that was a shame. Master Miura went on to study the more popular Sawada style after graduating from Yanagiya's school. Even when there is an opportunity to learn, the chance is lost unless one is eager to go after it.

GB-40 (kyū-kyo / qīu xū)

(VITAL AXIS): "Anterior and inferior to the external malleolus, in the middle of the depression."

(ILLUSTRATED): "In the depression, 0.3 unit in front of the inferior border of the external malleolus. In line with the fourth toe, three units above GB-41. In the biggest depression that forms when the toes are pushed into extension, with the foot slightly anteflexed. It is a place with a penetrating pain when pressed firmly with the fingertip."

LOCATION: In the depression anterior and inferior to the external malleolus (Fig. 2-83).

PALPATION: Flex and extend the ankle joint back and forth with one hand and use the thumb of the other hand to probe the depression in front of the external malleolus. Find the deepest part of the depression where there is tenderness.

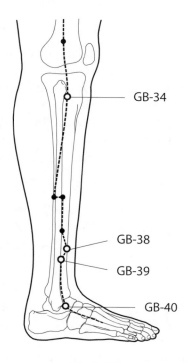

GB-34

GB-38

GB-39

GB-40

Fig. 2-83

INSERTION: Use a vertical or diagonal, superficial insertion with the needle pointed proximally.

INDICATION: I use GB-40 when there are imbalances in the Gallbladder meridian. It is especially useful when the Gallbladder meridian is excessive and there is a strong reaction at the point.

GB-39 (*ken-shō / xuán zhōng*)   ★★

(SYSTEMATIC): "Three units above the lateral malleolus, in the middle of the pulsation. [This is] the connecting point of the three yang meridians of the leg. Pressing [this] point stops the *yang ming* pulse. This means it is the right point."

(ILLUSTRATED): "On the lateral aspect of the lower leg three units above the lateral malleolus. Locate on the anterior margin of the tendon of the peroneus longus muscle. It is over the fibula where the muscle cannot be felt."

LOCATION: About four finger-widths above the lateral malleolus (Fig. 2-83).

PALPATION: To locate GB-39 on the right, I stand on the left side of the patient and grasp the right calf with my thumb on the Spleen meridian and the other four fingers on the Gallbladder meridian. I press with the tips of the four fingers, especially the middle finger, working my way downward toward the lateral malleolus from about two-thirds of the way down from the knee. Once I palpate the fibula, I move the fingers slightly posteriorly toward the Bladder meridian. I palpate a tight or tender point on the tendon by pressing in with the tip of the middle finger.

INSERTION: Use a vertical, shallow insertion. I usually do not retain the needle.

INDICATION: I use GB-39 to treat imbalances in the Gallbladder meridian, that is to say, I look for a reactive point between GB-34 and -40 for this purpose. When I want to disperse the Gallbladder meridian, I locate and needle the most reactive point along this line.

GB-38 (*yō-ho / yáng fŭ*)

(SYSTEMATIC): "Four units above the lateral malleolus, anterior to the fibula on the margin of the bone, about three-tenths of a unit in front. [It is] located seven units from GB-40."

(ILLUSTRATED): "On the lateral aspect of the calf, four units above the lateral malleolus. It is not on the line running straight down from GB-34, but instead is approximately a third of a unit anterior [to the line]. It is on the anterior margin of the tendon of the peroneus longus muscle."

LOCATION: On the vertical line below GB-34, on the anterior margin of the tendon of the peroneus longus muscle. GB-34 is found approximately one-third the distance up from the lateral malleolus to the bottom of the patella (Fig. 2-83).

PALPATION: Position yourself across from the leg you are going to palpate, as explained above for GB-39. Grasp the calf of the patient, who is lying prone, so that the thumb is on the medial side and the other four fingers are on the lateral side. Start working your way down from the midpoint between the head of the fibula and the lateral malleolus, pressing with the four fingers, especially the middle finger. When you find a hard spot, add a little back-and-forth (cross-fiber) movement to locate the exact point.

INSERTION: Use a vertical, shallow insertion, and do not retain the needle. Remove the needle as soon as the induration softens.

INDICATION: Primarily to disperse Gallbladder meridian excess.

DISCUSSION: In my practice, I find that imbalances in the Liver and Gallbladder meridians (felt in the left middle position of the pulse) are by far the most common. Usually, it is a Liver deficient/Gallbladder-excess pattern, and sometimes it is a Liver and Gallbladder excess pattern. The symptoms of medial knee pain, slight stifling sensation in the epigastrium or flank region, tension between GB-20 and GB-21, and pain or tension in the temples, are common in these patterns. In addition, I often find a tight band of tension running from GB-31 down to GB-34 or GB-38. Tonifying the yin meridian (at LR-3 or LR-8) and some dispersion (LR-2) is often enough to eliminate the excess palpated in the pulse, but sometimes this is not enough. Then it becomes necessary to disperse points on the Gallbladder meridian. When the right point is treated, the patient feels as if "a burden has been lifted" or that "an obstacle has been removed," to borrow the words of Inoue Keiri, one of the founders of meridian therapy.

GB-34 (*yō-ryō-sen* / *yáng líng quán*)

(*VITAL AXIS*): "In the depression lateral to the knee. Extend the knee to locate [this point]."

(*SYSTEMATIC*): "One unit below the knee, on the lateral margin of the fibula in the middle of the depression."

(*ILLUSTRATED*): "Below the head of the fibula is the tendon of the peroneus longus muscle, and [GB-34] is located on its anterior margin, anterior and inferior to the head of the fibula."

LOCATION: Anterior to the tendon, one finger-width below the head of the fibula (Fig. 2-83).

PALPATION: Press the tendon just below the head of the fibula with the tip of the thumb, and work your way down to find the tightest point on the tendon.

INSERTION: Shallow vertical insertion; do not retain the needle.

INDICATION: When there is marked tenderness, I use GB-34 to disperse excess in the Gallbladder meridian. GB-34 on the right is also useful for gallbladder diseases.

DISCUSSION: Sometimes when you compare the sensitivity of GB-34 on the right and left sides, there is a marked induration on the right side only. This indicates a possible gallbladder problem. Accordingly, I palpate the other diagnostic points for gallbladder dysfunction. There are two important points for diagnosis:

- Tenderness, induration, or sensitivity to pinching at ST-19 on the right
- Tenderness and induration medial to BL-19 on the right, next to the spinous process.

For both points, it is easy to tell if there is gallbladder dysfunction by pressing the same points on both sides and comparing their reactivity. Strong pressure sometimes causes an indescribable discomfort at GB-34 on the right. If all three diagnostic points for the gallbladder (GB-34, ST-19, and medial BL-19 on the right) are sensitive or reactive, cholecystitis (inflammation of the gallbladder) is very likely. Furthermore, if there is tenderness at GB-41 on the right, gallstones are likely (Gai, 1984). This method of assessment is described in the text *Acupuncture Point Diagnosis,* and I have found it to be quite accurate, especially concerning the likelihood of cholecystitis and the presence of positive findings at GB-34, ST-19, and medial BL-19 on the right. The reaction at all these gallbladder points indicates that cholecystitis is a result of Gallbladder excess. This may not be true in every single case, but there is a strong correlation. It follows that the treatment for cholecystitis consists of needling these reactive points.

Let me provide some more details about my technique. Rotation is applied to the needle after a shallow insertion in the right ST-19. After about a minute of stimulation, an intradermal needle is placed in this point, and retained. A needle is inserted about half a unit in the reactive point medial to BL-19 on the right. Then some rotation and gentle lifting and thrusting is applied. The needle is removed after about a minute, and five cones of direct moxibustion are applied. A needle is inserted about a third of a unit into the induration at GB-34 on the right. It is removed as soon as the induration softens. Of course, my treatment is not complete without a root treatment, so I usually tonify points like LR-8 or SP-2 first.

GB-30 *(kan-chō / huán tiào)*

(SYSTEMATIC): "It is on the middle of the greater trochanter. To locate [this point, have the patient] lie on the side and extend the leg on the bottom and flex the leg on top."

(HARA, 1807): "At the end of the crease [in the skin] when the top leg is flexed. [It is] below the bone in the depression where the finger fits in."

(ILLUSTRATED): "In the side-lying position, have the patient extend the bottom leg and flex the knee and hip joints of the top leg. Locate [this point] at the end of the crease which forms on the side of the hip joint."

LOCATION: At the end of the crease in the skin when the patient's hip is fully flexed (Fig. 2-84).

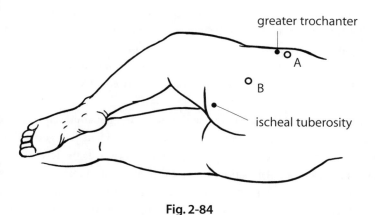

greater trochanter

A

B

ischeal tuberosity

Fig. 2-84

PALPATION: There are two possible locations.

- *Location A.* Find the tightest area on the side of the hip and press firmly with the middle finger. If the location of the tender point is not clear, try striking the

213

area with the knuckle of the little finger. This description is the standard Japanese location for GB-30.

- *Location B.* The more posterior location on the hip, which is the typical Chinese location for GB-30, can also be effective if the point is reactive. To locate this point, find a tight strand of muscle on the hip about four finger-widths posterior to the greater trochanter, then press with the fingertip to find the most tender or indurated point. Lightly striking this area sometimes produces a strong sensation that radiates to the anterior thigh.

INSERTION: Use a vertical insertion to a depth of one unit.

INDICATION: Again, the indication varies according to the point's location.

- *Location A.* Hip joint problems and leg pain; for some leg pain this is the only effective point.
- *Location B.* Pain in the lateral thigh around GB-31 and ST-32, as well as pain in the hip joint when Patrick's test[11] is negative.

DISCUSSION: Of the points on the hip, those around the Onodera point can be located and treated with the patient in a prone position. Points like GB-30 and the Gluteal point, however, are best treated with the patient in the side-lying position. Flexing the top leg at the hip and knee in the side-lying position extends the hip muscles and makes the points 'float' closer to the surface. This makes the point easier to locate and reach with a needle, and so shallow insertion suffices. Where it takes a 50- or 60mm needle to reach these points on the hip when the patient is prone, a 40mm needle is sufficient if the patient is in the side-lying position with the top leg flexed. Furthermore, it only takes a thin needle (No. 1 or 0) to get the desired response.

Also, when patients have acute sciatica with spontaneous pain, it is often impossible to get them to lie either supine or prone. So it is just good common sense to locate and treat points on the hips and legs as well as the lower back with the patient in the side-lying position. This is especially important when the needles are being retained and patients have to remain in that position for a while. However, be careful, because retaining needles in the local area in cases of acute sciatica can sometimes cause the pain to get worse. Pay attention to the patient's affected leg. When they have severe or spontaneous pain, they cannot help but move their legs a little from time to time. Also watch their face to see if they are grimacing. Of course, it is useful to ask the patient repeatedly during the treatment about the status of their pain.

Not just the treatment, but the examination and palpation of the lumbar area in the side-lying position is very useful as well. It is easier to press next to the spinous processes when approaching from above. And perhaps because the muscles around the waist tend to relax, you can find depressions right next to the spinous process-es, and these can be effective treatment points.

BL-67 *(shi-in / zhì yīn)*   ★

(SYSTEMATIC): "On the lateral side of the little toe, the width of a leek distant from the nail."

(ILLUSTRATED): "A tenth of a unit from the lateral base of the little toe. The finger comes to a stop at this point when pressing the base of the nail of the little toe with a fingernail."

LOCATION: Lateral to the nail of the little toe, 0.1 unit proximal to the corner of the nail (Fig. 2-85).

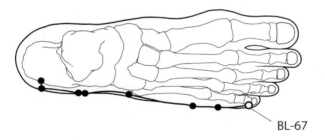

BL-67

Fig. 2-85

PALPATION: You will run into a wall when using the tip of your index finger to press distally toward the base of the toenail. The point is in the depression just next to the nail.

INSERTION: Only superficial insertion is possible.

INDICATION: I use BL-67 to tonify deficiency in the Bladder meridian. It is also useful for difficult labor and fetal malpresentation. Acupuncture works, but direct moxibustion is even more effective. I usually apply five cones on each side.

BL-60 (*kon-ron / kūn lún*) ★

(SYSTEMATIC): "Behind the lateral malleolus; in the depression above the calcaneus. A small pulsation can be felt here."

(ILLUSTRATED): "Posterior to the lateral malleolus on the anterior border of the Achilles tendon; in the depression above the calcaneus."

LOCATION: In the depression at the midpoint between the lateral malleolus and the Achilles tendon (Fig. 2-86).

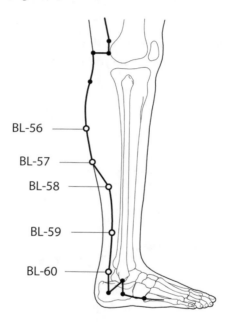

BL-56

BL-57

BL-58

BL-59

BL-60

Fig. 2-86

PALPATION: When locating BL-60 with the patient prone, grab the foot with one hand and move the ankle into plantar flexion. Place the thumb of the other hand just above the calcaneus, between the lateral malleolus and the Achilles tendon. Bend the distal joint of the thumb in a right angle, and press in a posterior direction to the calcaneus with the tip of the thumb as you move it back and forth (in a cross-fiber motion) to locate an indurated or tender point. BL-60 can also be located with the ankle in dorsiflexion. For this, use the tip of the middle finger to probe in the depression between the lateral malleolus and the Achilles tendon with a circular motion.

INSERTION: Diagonal insertion with the needle pointing posteriorly and downward. Insert just to a depth where the tip of the needle reaches the induration.

INDICATION: I use BL-60 to treat imbalances in the Bladder meridian. I usually use BL-60 for dispersion. In terms of symptoms, it is effective for occipital headaches and pain in either the upper or lower back.

BL-59 *(fu-yō / fū yáng)*

(SYSTEMATIC): "Three units above the lateral malleolus. Anterior to the *tai yang* [meridian] and posterior to the *shao yang* [meridian]. In the space between bone and muscle."

(ILLUSTRATED): "Three units superior to [the highest point of] the lateral malleolus; on the anterior margin of the Achilles tendon."

LOCATION: Three units superior to the lateral malleolus on the posterior margin of the fibula (Fig. 2-86).

PALPATION: Slide a fingertip proximally along the margin of the fibula from BL-60 (behind the lateral malleolus). There will be a puffy place about three units above the malleolus. Press the posterior aspect of the fibula with the tip of the thumb to locate a tender point. When there is no reaction, try palpating closer to the Achilles tendon.

INSERTION: Use a vertical, superficial insertion.

INDICATION: Sciatica and lower back pain

DISCUSSION: Active acupuncture points are interesting things. Just by lightly stroking over them with the pad of a finger, you can tell something is there. To borrow an expression from the first chapter of *Vital Axis*, "The guest is at the gate." By stroking over the point, one detects a slight depression or otherwise some puffiness or tension. In the latter case, the "guest" is an unwanted one known as a pathogenic influence *(jaki/xié qì)*. At BL-59, the latter case is the most common. One often feels as if there is some fluid retention right around the point. This stagnation of fluids is sometimes called 'fluid poison' *(sui doku/shuǐ dú)*. When there is nothing like puffiness or a swollen spot, and the area feels just like the margin of a bone, then there is no guest at the gate. Of course, acupuncture and moxibustion would be ineffective in this case. We must look for a reaction at other points, such as BL-58 or BL-60. This type of reaction (puffiness) occurs at other points on the margin of bones, such as SP-6.

The point that feels puffy when stroked is often also very sensitive to pinching, and sometimes the patient will jump. Pressing the point can also be very painful for the patient. The reaction can vary, and is often indicative of the underlying pathology (Table 2-2).

Pathology	Reaction
The condition of the epidermis has changed	Can be detected just by stroking the point
The condition of the subcutaneous and fatty tissues is different	When there is sensitivity to pinching
The condition of the fascia and superficial muscle tissue is affected	When there is pain with pressure (tenderness)

Table 2-2

BL-59 is a unique point in that quite often there is a reaction in all three layers. Most points tend to be tender but not sensitive to pinching, or vice versa. In this sense, BL-59 is effective no matter the depth of the needle insertion.

My location for BL-59, by the way, is a little different from most texts. In the classics, of which *Systematic Classic of Acupuncture and Moxibustion* is representative, BL-59 is located "in the space between [the] bone and muscle," which is to say, in the middle, between the Achilles tendon and the fibula. In *Illustrated Manual to Practical Acupuncture and Moxibustion Points,* Honma located BL-59 "on the anterior margin of the Achilles tendon," that is, next to the Achilles tendon. My location is right next to the fibula. So it is closer to the Gallbladder meridian. Comparing these three locations in my practice, I find that the reaction appears in the following order of frequency:

next to the bone > in the middle > next to the tendon

Some time ago, I woke up suddenly in the middle of the night with a cramp in my right leg. It was not a spasm in the gastrocnemius muscle. Rather, it was a cramp in the lateral thigh from the knee up to the hip joint. The pain was intense and my cry woke up my wife as well as our dog, who started barking. I always have needles by my bedside. Placing and retaining needles in GB-30 and BL-59 relieved the spasm.

BL-59 is an indispensable point for spontaneous pain in the lower back, hip, and leg (sciatica). Often, it is difficult to lie in the supine or prone position when there is severe pain in the back or hips. In such cases, I palpate BL-59 with the patient lying on the unaffected side. Sometimes just pressing the point relieves the pain. When this happens, you know the point will be effective, and the moment the needle is inserted, the pain diminishes or disappears. BL-59 is remarkably effective for sciatica, and this is no doubt related to it being the cleft point of the Yang Heel vessel *(yō kyō myaku/yáng qiāo mài)*.

On the other hand, sometimes when treating spontaneous pain in the leg and hip, the pain becomes worse right after a needle is inserted in BL-59, or after it is retained for a while. This is especially true for acute cases of sciatica, so one has to be careful.

Once I got a call from a novice practitioner who was at a loss as to how to treat a case of severe sciatica. He had talked to the senior instructor of our study group who told him he needed to check the pulse carefully and treat the patient according to the pattern. However, obviously, this man was looking for quick results—he wanted to know how to obtain symptomatic relief. The correct way to do meridian therapy is to examine the pulse and abdomen, and then look for active points, starting with tonification points. Symptomatic treatment comes only after the root treatment, so it is nearly impossible to do a treatment just to stop the pain. However, this is the orthodox approach, and there are other ways to go about a treatment—the back door as opposed to the front entrance. Before I started practicing meridian therapy, I went through the back door all the time. Therefore, I suggested the following strategy.

With the patient lying on the unaffected side, palpate the most reactive point around BL-59. Insert a needle shallowly in the reactive point and retain the needle. If the pain starts to get worse, remove the needle immediately and switch to direct moxibustion on the same point. Keep applying cones there until the pain disappears or subsides. Continue with the direct moxibustion at least until the pain is not as bad as it was when the patient came in. There will be some measure of relief after 30 to 50 cones. In this way, you must use each point as if it was the only one. Do not give in to the temptation to use many points, and especially avoid retaining too many needles. Use a maximum of five points. If treating just BL-59 is enough to make the spontaneous pain disappear, call it a day. It may seem like this is not enough treatment, but the initial effect of treating BL-59 will diminish as you stimulate more points. This is called 'killing the effect of a point'. You will get good results using more points only if you needle each point with the utmost care using a noninsertive technique.

It was several days later that the man to whom I gave this advice called me back to thank me. It seems that this approach worked well for him, but actually, lessons like this are best learned when you confront difficulties in the clinic yourself and arrive at a solution through a process of trial and error. Figuring things out on one's own, however, is not very common in this day and age. There is a lack of courage and fortitude, especially when one enters this profession after reaching middle age. Novice practitioners tend to look for a safe and sure way. This is to be expected.

More than twenty-five years ago, when I was young and struggling to get a practice going, I went on a house call to treat a woman who was over thirty-years old. She was a vegetable farmer, and she had become immobilized with pain while working in a greenhouse. I found her lying on the ground on her side among cucumber plants. Her left hip was in so much pain that she could not move. As soon as I inserted a needle in BL-59, the spontaneous pain stopped. I then tried to get her to move, but movement was still difficult because of the pain. So I inserted another needle in the Iliac point on the left, and then she was able to get up with only moderate pain. Of course, we were both relieved and elated. This woman still comes for treatment from time to time. We laugh as we say how our hair and faces betray our age despite how young we feel. I have many such memorable episodes with BL-59.

BL-58 (*hi-yō / fēi yáng*)   ★★★

(*SYSTEMATIC*): "Seven units above the lateral malleolus. [It is] the connecting point of the *tai yang* [meridian] of the leg and [here it] separates to [go to] the *shao yang* [meridian]. In the space between bone and muscle."

(*ILLUSTRATED*): "Seven units superior to the lateral malleolus. By applying pressure and stroking upward on the anterior margin of the Achilles tendon, you run into the lateral head of the gastrocnemius muscle. BL-58 is lateral and slightly inferior to BL-57 [where the heads of the gastrocnemius separate]."

220

LOCATION: One-fourth of the way up from the lateral malleolus to the knee (patella), on the posterior margin of the fibula (Fig. 2-86).

PALPATION: With the tip of the thumb, press the space between the posterior margin of the fibula and the anterior margin of the Achilles tendon. Move the thumb proximally in this groove to find a tender point one-fifth to one-fourth of the way up toward the knee. This point location varies a great deal, so do not be too concerned with standard measurements.

INSERTION: Use a diagonal, superficial insertion with the needle tip aimed anteriorly behind the fibula.

INDICATION: I use BL-58 for imbalances in the Bladder meridian. It is also effective for pain and tension in the occiput, lower back and leg pain, as well as paralysis.

DISCUSSION: As with BL-59, I locate BL-58 quite differently from the standard method in the textbooks. The trick is to locate the point right next to the fibula. If there is no reaction next to the bone, then I look more toward the gastrocnemius. Therefore, my BL-58 ends up somewhere between the Bladder and Gallbladder meridians.

    The indication for BL-58 is almost the same as BL-59 except that BL-58 is more effective in correcting imbalances in the Bladder meridian. The superiority of BL-58 in this respect is no doubt due to its being the connecting point. BL-58 is also ideal for home moxibustion treatments for lower back pain or sciatica. This point should be located with the patient in the side-lying position since the moxibustion can be done in a similar position by the patient's friend or family member.

BL-56 (shō-kin / chéng jīn)

(SYSTEMATIC): "In the middle of the calf muscle in the depression."

(ILLUSTRATED): "Five units below BL-40. Palpate the most prominent part of the gastrocnemius muscle, and locate [the point] in the groove of the muscle between the lateral and medial heads."

LOCATION: In the middle of the gastrocnemius muscle, between the lateral and medial heads (Fig. 2-86).

PALPATION: Press the center of the gastrocnemius muscle with the tip of the middle finger and move it up and down to find the depression. There is a point in the depression that is tender with slight pressure. Sometimes this point is more distal, closer to BL-57.

INSERTION: Use a vertical, superficial insertion.

INDICATION: Spasms in the gastrocnemius muscle.

DISCUSSION: When you grab the calf muscle of a patient who suffers from calf spasms or shin splints, the side that usually gets the spasms is harder than the other side. It sometimes feels as if the entire muscle is hardened. This tends to occur in patients with problems in the leg, such as arthritis in the knee, sciatica, or arteritis (inflammation of an artery). When the calf muscle on the affected side begins to soften, it is a sign that such problems are beginning to resolve.

BL-40 (*i-chū* / *wěi zhōng*)   ★★

(SYSTEMATIC): "In the middle of the crease [in the back] of the knee, on the pulsation."

(ILLUSTRATED): "In the middle of the popliteal fossa where there is a pulsation."

LOCATION: The point is located in the middle of the popliteal fossa (Fig. 2-87).

PALPATION: Find the crease in the back of the knee by flexing the knee a little. Then palpate the most indurated or tender point on the crease.

INSERTION: Use a vertical, shallow insertion.

INDICATION: Knee pain, lower back pain.

DISCUSSION: A reaction appears at BL-40 whenever there is knee pain, especially when the range of motion in the knee joint is reduced (Table 2-3).

Walking becomes difficult when the range of motion in the knee joint is greatly reduced; in such cases, walking causes pain. In advanced cases like this, a hard knot forms in the muscle in the vicinity of BL-40. Acupuncture alone is not sufficient to deal with this induration. I recommend direct moxibustion treatments at home. There are not that many people these days who are skillful at applying direct moxibustion, but this actually works in their favor in this case. Creating burns on the induration at BL-40 can sometimes bring surprising results. Larger cones of

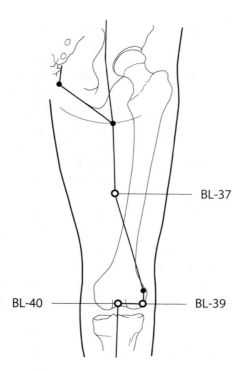

Fig. 2-87

Pathology	Reaction
In osteoarthritis of the knee with genu varum (also known as *bowleg*)	Usually appears on the medial aspect of the knee
In osteoarthritis of the knee with genu valgum (also known as *knock knee*)	Usually appears on the lateral aspect of the knee
When there is flexion deformity in the knee	In the popliteal fossa, especially around BL-40

Table 2-3

direct moxibustion work not only for flexion deformity, but for all types of osteo-arthritis of the knee.

I have known for a long time that large cones were better in cases of frozen shoulders, but more recently I have found that this applies also to knee problems. Now I recommend large cones of direct moxibustion for these conditions as long as there is no obvious inflammation in the joint and the joint does not feel espe-cially warm. When there is inflammation, I either retain an intradermal needle or recommend small cones of direct moxibustion. Direct moxibustion on BL-40 is the best treatment for flexion deformity, but BL-40 also happens to be one of the most sensitive points. It takes a lot of resolve to undertake this moxibustion treatment at home.

I saw a woman in her fifties with flexion deformity and genu valgum in her left knee. She had spontaneous pain at night and the medial aspect of her knee was swollen and warm to the touch. A closer examination revealed that she also had a mild case of sciatica in her left leg. Treatments using BL-59 and the Ischeal point relieved the pain at night, and home moxibustion treatments on BL-40, ST-34, M-LE-16, and ST-40 gradually reduced the deformity. The patient was pleased with the improvement because the reduction in the deformity made it easier to walk. Her condition improved even more than I expected, and the surgery that had been recommended became unnecessary. Actually, this patient had come for a few treat-ments a year before when her condition was not as serious. As soon as her pain was relieved, instead of persisting to obtain full recovery, she stopped coming for treat-ment. Even after the pain recurred, she avoided coming in again, using the excuses that moxibustion was painful and old-fashioned, and my clinic was too far away. Her condition became steadily worse so she went to an orthopedist who gave her shots and extracted fluid from her swollen knee joint. As her knee continued to worsen, she finally relented and came back to my clinic for treatment. Now that she is doing so much better, she has promised to continue with her home moxibustion regimen.

I have experienced several cases like this where remarkable results were obtained by persistent moxibustion treatment at home. In every case, the patients apply larg-er cones of moxibustion than I suggested. In these cases, larger cones seem to work in their favor. I am convinced now, more than ever, that direct moxibustion has almost miraculous effects that are different from those obtained with acupuncture. After all, historically, many practitioners in Japan have treated serious diseases with moxibustion alone. I myself recovered from tuberculosis, pleuritis, and peritonitis with repeated moxibustion treatments. This is why I maintain that direct moxibus-tion is the most fundamental treatment for knee problems.

BL-39 (*i-yō / wěi yáng*)

(SYSTEMATIC): "Lateral to the *tai yang* meridian of the leg and posterior to the *shao yang* meridian, [this point] emerges on the lateral margin of the popliteal fossa between two tendons."

(ILLUSTRATED): "On the lateral margin of the popliteal fossa, two units lateral to BL-40. It is located medial to the thick tendon of the biceps femoris muscle."

LOCATION: Lateral to BL-40 and medial to the tendon and the bone (Fig. 2-87).

PALPATION: An induration or tender point can be found when pressing the lateral margin of the popliteal fossa toward the bone with the tip of the thumb.

INSERTION: Use a vertical, shallow insertion.

INDICATION: Lower back pain, sciatica.

DISCUSSION: Baba Hakkō, one of the old guards of meridian therapy, does not use many symptomatic points in his treatments. He mostly does a thorough root treatment, taking the pulses, needling the five-phasic points, and taking the pulses again. I observed a treatment of his at a seminar where he eliminated the lower back pain of one patient with simple insertion in BL-39. I tried this technique right away on a patient of mine who came in with acute lower back pain. I succeeded in alleviating his pain without using any points on his back by needling only five-phasic points on his leg. My success was short-lived, however, because as soon as he walked out my door, he doubled over as the pain returned. So you cannot always count on techniques that are new to you. Nowadays I usually use BL-40, and limit BL-39 to those situations when there is back or knee pain and it is more reactive than BL-40.

BL-37 (*in-mon / yīn mén*)

(SYSTEMATIC): "Six units under the cleft in the flesh [BL-36 or the gluteal crease]."

(ILLUSTRATED): "In the midpoint between BL-36 and 40."

LOCATION: In the center of the posterior thigh, slightly above the midpoint between the gluteal crease and the popliteal fossa (Fig. 2-87).

PALPATION: The hamstrings soften when the foot is lifted off the table (slight flexion of knee) in a patient who is lying prone. Probe with the middle finger using a back-and-forth motion to find an induration. It can be found in the middle of a tight strand of muscle. Locate the hardest point.

INSERTION: Use a vertical, shallow insertion.

INDICATION: Sciatica, stiffness in legs.

DISCUSSION: Those who work in a standing position under tension, such as carpenters and masons, often get chronic tension in their hamstrings. Inserting a thin needle in an induration around BL-37 brings wonderful relief for patients like this. In such cases, it is also a good idea to relieve the hardness and tenderness in points around the Onodera point.

Ischeal point *(den-chō / tún dǐng)*   ★★★

LOCATION: Over the ischeal tuberosity (Fig. 2-88).

PALPATION: The Ischeal point must be located with the patient in the side-lying position, just as with the Gluteal point. Therefore, the leg on the bottom is extended and the hip joint of the top leg must be flexed at least 90°. The knee of the top leg must rest on the table so that the patient is stable. It is also possible to rest the knee on a pillow or bolster. Locate the ischeal tuberosity and strike it lightly to see if it is tender. I use the knuckle of my little finger. If there is tenderness with striking, press the point with the tip of your middle finger using a circular motion to find the most tender point.

INSERTION: Use a vertical insertion toward the ischeal tuberosity. I use a 40mm, No. 0 needle, and usually insert approximately half the length of the needle (2cm). I sometimes insert up to one unit (3cm) for obese patients.

INDICATION: Sciatica.

DISCUSSION: Since there is a Gluteal point, which covers indurations and tender points on the gluteus, perhaps one would think that there is no need to designate a separate point over the ischeal tuberosity. After treating many patients with sciatica, however, I have come to the conclusion that this point over the ischeal tuberosity is decidedly different from others in the gluteal region. I therefore decided to introduce it as a miscellaneous point here at the end of the chapter.

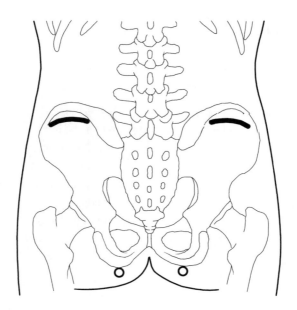

Fig. 2-88

To locate the point, the patient must be in the side-lying position, with the hip joint on the top flexed. This brings the ischeal tuberosity closer to the surface. The sciatic nerve also comes closer to the surface, so a 40mm needle is long enough if the patient is in the side-lying position.

To test for a reaction, use percussion or a strike at the point. This technique takes a little practice, but striking lightly with the knuckle of the little finger is a quick way to find out if there are tender points. Even the hardness of the underlying tissue can be felt. When an inexperienced person tries striking this point, the patient often says "No, that's not the place." Practice makes all the difference.

Treatment at this point requires the use of a thin needle. It is difficult to feel the arrival of qi with a thick needle, so I use a No. 0 needle. A strong *dé qì* sensation is not needed here.

It is possible to locate and treat the Ischeal point with the patient in a prone position, but it is harder to find and needle. One must use a 50- or 60mm needle to reach the point when the patient is prone. This reduces the chances of getting the needle to the right point. In any case, along with the Gluteal point just above it, the Ischeal point is highly effective when there is a marked reaction.

Onodera point (*Onodera-shi attsu-ten*)

This point was discovered by a Japanese physician named Naosuke Onodera as an indication of peptic ulcers. It is more a reactive area than a point.

(*NANZANDŌ MEDICAL DICTIONARY, 1978*): "This point is palpated with the patient in the side-lying position with the [top] leg flexed at the hip and knee; the practitioner applies strong pressure toward the bone with a fingertip on points three to four centimeters below the iliac crest. The line of palpation below the iliac crest is divided into three sections: anterior, middle, and posterior. These indicate, respectively, pathology in the (a) esophagus, (b) cardia [upper part of stomach], and (c) the remainder of the stomach and duodenum. Usually both sides are equally tender, but it is said that tenderness is stronger on the left side when there is a gastric ulcer, and on the right side when there is a duodenal ulcer."

LOCATION: In the gluteal muscles about 5cm below the iliac crest (Fig. 2-88).

INSERTION: I locate this point with the patient lying prone. Gently press points about 5cm below the iliac crest, starting from the anterior superior iliac spine and working toward the posterior superior iliac spine. An induration is usually found somewhere in the middle. Press the induration firmly with a fingertip while applying small circular motions to locate the hardest point.

The Onodera point is actually more difficult to locate when the patient is lying on the side. In addition, it is rare, but it does happen, that indurations appear all along the horizontal line inferior to the iliac crest. Treat only the hardest point. Reactions along the Onodera zone appear across a broad area, and they change quickly, that is, the indurations move with the treatment. It therefore takes skill to locate and treat this area.

INSERTION: Use a diagonal, deep insertion with the needle tip pointing toward the foot. Insert 30- to 50mm, as if you were attempting to penetrate the induration. The insertion should be deeper for obese patients.

INDICATION: Pain in the leg and the hip joint, fatigue in the posterior thigh, and diseases of the upper gastrointestinal tract

DISCUSSION: There seems to be a specific pattern in the way reactive points appear in cases of lower back and leg pain (Table 2-4). These patterns can be used for both diagnosis and treatment.

Pathology	Reaction
In L1 to L3 and in the femoral cutaneous nerve	Around GB-30
In L4 to L5 and in the sciatic nerve	At the Gluteal point or Ischeal point
Other types of leg pain and hip joint pathology	At the Onodera point

Table 2-4

I do not use the Onodera point for sciatica or myofascial lower back pain. I find the Onodera point is reactive (tender or indurated) in patients who strain their legs, for example, carpenters, those who work on steep hills, and people with curved backs who have to tense their legs to maintain their balance. Stiffness in the hips and hamstrings is often immediately relieved by needling or applying direct moxibustion on the Onodera point.

A 55-year-old woman once came for treatment because she was unable to walk due to severe pain in her left lower back and leg. She almost had to be lifted onto the treatment table by two helpers who accompanied her. In addition to the lower back and leg pain, she had deformity and arthritic pain in her left knee and ankle. I palpated a large induration that was extremely tender at the left Onodera point. I inserted a 50mm, No. 3 needle into the tightest point and retained the needle for about ten minutes. I applied fifteen cones of direct moxibustion on the point after removing the needle. Since her pattern was Spleen deficiency, I also needled SP-3, CV-12, and CV-14. At the end of the treatment, the patient was able to get off the table and walk without assistance.

Soon after she got home, she called to say how thrilled she was that the spontaneous pain in her hip and leg were gone. She has continued to come in for occasional treatments in the two years since. Her condition has steadily improved, and the induration at the Onodera point is gone. When I press deeply in the area, however, I can feel a soft lumpy strand of muscle next to the bone, and this is still useful as a treatment point.

ENDNOTES

1. Shanghai College of Traditional Medicine, *Acupuncture: A Comprehensive Text*. Chicago: Eastland Press, 1981: 336.

2. The distal five-phasic points—*sei/jǐng, ei/yíng, yu/shū, kei/jīng,* and *gō/hé*—are most literally translated as well, gushing, transporting, traversing, and uniting. However, the more commonly known names for these points—well, spring, stream, river, and sea—are used in this text.

3. The *sōmyaku/zōng mài* area is a place where many channels and vessels converge around the Lungs. This term is also translated as pectoral vessels.

4. Also known as *san ou sha shin tō/sān huáng xiè xīn tāng,* this formula consists of Rhizoma Copitidis *(ou ren/huáng lián),* Radix Scutellariae *(ou kin/huáng qín),* and Radix et Rhizoma Rhei *(dai ou/dà huáng).*

5. Orthostatic albuminuria is a type of benign proteinuria seen occasionally in young people. This form of proteinuria appears when standing but disappears when lying down, and it does not appear at night when one is sleeping. It is thought to be caused by a weak constitution with excessive lumbar lordosis that presses on the renal vein, causing congestion.

6. The hyperabduction syndrome is seen with conditions such as osteoarthritis of the cervical spine where strong abduction of the upper arm exacerbates the pain, induces paresthesia, and compromises circulation in the arm. One characteristic is the loss of the radial pulse with strong abduction of the upper arm.

7. The issue of local treatment versus distal treatment is discussed under point ST-19.

8. *Senki (shàn qì)* is also known as *sho-cho ki-tsu (xiǎo chǎng qì tòng)* and refers to hernias, urogenital diseases, and severe pain in the lower abdomen with constipation and oliguria. In Japan *senki* became a general category of male urogenital disease which includes everything from kidney stones to inguinal hernias.

9. The Japan Meridian and Points Committee was formed at the International Conference of Acupuncture held in Tokyo in 1965. Under the auspices of the WHO, this committee has worked with representatives from other countries to standardize the names and numbers of acupuncture points.

10. Some practitioners refer to this point as Posterior LR-13.

11. Patrick's test consists of the following: With the patient in a supine position, the hip and knee are flexed. Then the external malleolus is placed over the patella of the opposite leg, and the knee is depressed. Arthritis of the hip is indicated if pain is produced by this test.

CHAPTER THREE

Effectively Treating
Acupuncture Points

My Approach to Treatment

THE REASON WE ACUPUNCTURISTS make such a fuss over acupuncture points is simply because we want to improve our clinical results. No matter how we play around with the idea of point location, if it does not serve to relieve our patients' symptoms and improve their health, it is nothing more than a mind game. Table 3-1 shows the factors that influence the clinical outcome.

---

1. Which points are needled (procedure for point selection): looking, listening, questioning, pulse diagnosis, abdominal diagnosis, meridian palpation (tender points, indurations, depressions, skin temperature, pinching diagnosis, percussion)

2. Which points are emphasized:

    A. points receiving primary emphasis — 1 to 3 points
    B. points receiving secondary emphasis — up to 7 points
    C. all other points — 10+ points

Table 3-1

Assuming that we needle twenty points in a whole body treatment, it is possible to categorize the level of emphasis as shown in the table. Even when the number of points used in a treatment is significantly greater or less than twenty, the number of primary points (category A) does not change substantially, while the number of points belonging to categories B and C can be modified as necessary.

This means that we put everything we have into category A points, using one point for the root treatment and one or possibly two points for symptomatic treatment. In acupuncture treatments there is no need to put the same amount of effort into each and every point. Knowing how to vary the emphasis or intensity is just as important in acupuncture as it is in good acting and for life in general. Proper emphasis simply leaves a better impression. People like to receive acupuncture from an experienced practitioner, but even then, there are times when it seems as if something is missing in their treatment. It is often just a lack of emphasis. Patients are likely to go home more satisfied when just two or three points are highlighted.

Needles and Techniques

There is a great deal that can be said about the techniques of Japanese acupuncture and moxibustion. Describing all the techniques in detail, however, is beyond the scope of this book. You can refer to my first book *Japanese Classical Acupuncture: Introduction to Meridian Therapy* (Shudo, 1990) for specific instructions on needling using an insertion tube. Also *Japanese Acupuncture* by Birch and Ida (1998) is an excellent resource for learning the techniques of Japanese acupuncture and moxibustion. In this section, I will present a brief outline of the needles[1] I use and the depths of insertion, followed by a brief explanation of various techniques. In the section that follows, I will discuss what I consider to be the most important aspect of needling—the "arrival of qi" *(ki itaru/zhì qì)*.

Table 3-2 lists the various needles and their common usages while Table 3-3 lists the needling depths. The details supplied in Tables 3-2 and 3-3 form the basis for the various techniques I use during treatment—contact needling, simple insertion, retaining the needle, intradermal needling—and these are discussed in greater detail below. There is also a discussion of direct moxibustion, another essential aspect of my treatments.

- *Contact needling.* In this technique, the needle is rotated with the tip resting on the skin. No attempt is made to insert the needle, but sometimes the needle does

Needle	Usage
5mm No. 0 or 1 (intradermal needle)	Horizontal superficial insertion
30mm No. 02 or 01	Tonification and superficial insertion
40mm No. 1	Dispersion and shallow insertion
50mm No. 3	Deep insertion
60mm No. 3	Especially deep points on the lumbar and hip

Table 3-2

Mode of insertion	Depth (mm)
Contact needling *(sesshoku-shin)*	0
Super-superficial insertion *(chōsenshi)*	0.5
Superficial insertion *(seppi-shin)*	1 to 3
Shallow insertion *(senshi)*	4 to 10
Deep insertion *(shinshi)*	10 to 50

Table 3-3

work its way about a millimeter under the skin. I call this super-superficial inser-tion. Technically, it is the same as contact needling. This technique is useful for deficient patients with fatigue, depression, loss of motivation, and psychosomat-ic conditions. I also use it exclusively on children, and on patients who dislike needle sensation, as well as those who have a fever or are sweating. Super-super-ficial insertion is effective for spontaneous pain and lower back pain with move-ment in elderly women (osteoarthritis and osteoporosis). I also use this technique when treating tinnitus with points around the ear, like TB-20, because insertion can make the tinnitus worse.

• *Simple insertion.* In this technique, the needle is inserted but not retained. I use this technique in every situation where contact needling or retaining the needle is not necessary. I tend to use simple insertion especially for root treatment points.

• *Retaining the needle.* I used to retain many needles as long as the patient was not overly sensitive. In recent years, however, I have reduced the number of needles I retain. These days I retain a needle when a point is especially reactive and is connected to the patient's main complaint, and I want to get the maximum effect out of that point. Sometimes, for the root treatment, I will retain a needle in a tonification point on one side to extend the effect of tonification. Needless to say, needles should be retained only in patients who are not hypersensitive or especially deficient.

• *Intradermal needling.* I use intradermal needles to increase and extend the effect of a treatment. I place an intradermal needle in just one point at a time. I try intradermal needles on chronic pain cases when the symptom does not improve, placing an intradermal needle in the most painful or excessive point.

There are certain situations where I routinely use intradermal needles. The first is for vertigo. I retain an intradermal needle in the auricular vertigo point, which is a tender point in the occipitomastoid junction on the more reactive side. The second is for motion sickness, where I retain an intradermal needle in KI-9 on both sides. The third is SP-6, which I use when there is a possibility of a gynecological problem and when the point is very tender. Finally, I use intradermal needles in a reactive axillary point on one side for asthma or coughing, or on the left side in cases of heart disease.

• *Direct moxibustion.* There has been a long tradition of moxibustion in Japan, and direct moxibustion stands on its own as a highly effective modality. I provide direct moxibustion in my practice to extend the effect of the acupuncture treatment. It is especially useful to have patients learn to apply direct moxibustion themselves at home on the points I indicate. I tend to use more direct moxibustion for chronic musculoskeletal conditions, such as osteoarthritis, which do not respond as quickly to acupuncture. I begin with a small dose of three sesame seed-sized cones on each point for children or very depleted patients. The standard dose is five half-rice-grain-sized cones on each point. Aside from this, there are special points that require multiple cones (from 20 to 50 half-rice-grain-sized cones) to be effective.

The Arrival of Qi

The ability to feel and facilitate the arrival of qi is important for giving effective acupuncture treatment. I am sure there are other practitioners with different techniques, but I have my own for facilitating the arrival of qi. Not much is written about this subject, perhaps because it is not so easy to explain. There are, however, references to the arrival of qi in the earliest classics. It is described in the first chapter of *Vital Axis* as follows:

> The important thing about acupuncture is that the effect comes with the arrival of qi. The sign of this is like the wind blowing the clouds away. It becomes clear and bright, like looking into the blue sky.

This passage aptly describes how it feels when the symptom clears after the arrival of qi. The arrival of qi is synonymous with the needle having an effect.

People often ask me what the arrival of qi feels like. Yanagiya Sorei, the man who revived traditional acupuncture in Japan, explained it this way:

> The coming and going of qi is described in the classics as (1) a feeling of heaviness or tension, (2) pulsation, (3) some trembling, (4) a floating feeling, (5) a sinking feeling, (6) heaviness or dampness, (7) sensation of heat, (8) a refreshing coolness, and (9) spontaneous movement in the needle. When the practitioner is able to feel the coming and going of qi like this in his inserting or supporting hand, he can be considered to be a full-fledged acupuncturist. (Yanagiya, 1980)

Yanagiya also used the analogy of fishing:

> The needle tip coming into contact with skin can be likened to a fishhook with bait contacting the surface of the water. The moment of contact, it feels as if the fish has taken the bait, as if the fish has swallowed the hook. Then it feels like the hook sinks under the water with the weight of the lead. [Thus the needle] breaks the skin, goes through the fascia, penetrates the muscle fibers, and runs into a tendon or ligament. Then it feels like the lead weight on the line hits the bottom. Acupuncture feels exactly like fishing. When it feels like [the needle is in] tofu, gradually it begins to feel heavier as the needle is inserted. Thus, the flesh begins to tighten [around the needle], or the fish gets caught on the hook. This is called the arrival of qi. The feeling of [the tissue] where the needle has been inserted can be sensed in the [inserting] hand which holds the needle. This sensation enables one to know the condition of the body where the needle has been inserted. (Yanagiya, 1977)

My experience of the arrival of qi is that, as I insert the needle, it begins to feel heavier, as if something were slowly closing in around it. After a while, it begins to feel like I am needling a piece of leather. It is not so good if the needle goes in without resistance. There has to be resistance, as if something was preventing the advance of the needle. Sometimes muscle fibers actually wrap around the needle and it becomes stuck, but this is not what I am talking about. The arrival of qi is characterized by free movement of the needle along with a feeling of resistance at its tip.

This sensation in the needle is felt by the practitioner, and it is a pleasant sensation that is hard to describe. It does not matter whether the patient feels something or not. Once you feel the arrival of qi, it is enough.

Often, when I feel the arrival of qi, my mouth fills with saliva. Quite often the patient will report feeling a pleasant sensation as well. Some nod in agreement, and others say "Yes! That's it! That's the place." Patients are sometimes surprised to learn that I am also aware of their sensation. I tell them "Of course! This is my business."

Some people confuse the arrival of qi with *tokki/dé qì*, which is a needle sensation that the patient feels. The arrival of qi is felt first by the practitioner, and again, it does not matter whether the patient feels it or not. Both the arrival of qi *(zhì qì)* and obtaining qi *(dé qì)* are terms used in *Basic Questions*. In Japan today, these two terms are generally understood to mean two different things. In any case, most practitioners who feel the arrival of qi feel some sensation of tingling, warmth, or pulsation in their inserting or supporting hand. I would like to relate a little of my own experience.

Learning to Feel the Arrival of Qi

It has been forty years since I first opened my acupuncture practice. Thinking back, it seems like it was after about twenty-five years of practice that I started to get a feel for the arrival of qi. It was only after thirty years that I became sure about the feeling. That is how long it took me, and it is nothing to be proud of. However, once you recognize the arrival of qi, you know whether an insertion is effective or not, and you gain confidence in your treatments. Also, giving treatments starts to become fun. It does take time, however, to get a feel for the arrival of qi.

People ask me how they can learn to feel the arrival of qi, and whether this feeling is necessary for effective treatment. It takes daily practice to become a full-fledged acupuncturist. If you keep the arrival of qi in mind each time you insert a needle, eventually you will begin to feel it. How long it will take is hard to say. It could take as long as thirty years, like me, or perhaps ten or just five years. I think this ability can be acquired even faster by those who make a special effort, or those who are creative or have natural ability. Even so, it is realistic to think in terms of five to ten years. My answer to those students who cannot wait that long and want to acquire this skill right away, is "Perhaps you should give up acupuncture and try another profession." Becoming a skilled acupuncturist requires that much dedication.

Yanagiya (1980) observed:

> Inserting needles and applying moxa, this is an art. Ours is a profession which requires a sense of adventure. Isn't it incredible how all manner of diseases can be cured with nothing more than a needle or a few pieces of moxa? Isn't it grand how needles and moxa can be used to create the effect of all manner of medicine?
>
> Acupuncture is of the mind. This should be considered very carefully. One needle can be used to unlock the key to all manner of diseases. It is only natural, therefore, that one's technique needs to be perfected.

Acupuncture is a profession in which we use a thin piece of wire in an attempt to cure conditions which do not respond to medicines. Without a doubt, this is an extremely challenging profession. So it requires a continual refinement of technique. I feel indescribable joy in having this profession in which I can demonstrate my finesse.

How to Induce the Arrival of Qi

The importance of the arrival of qi should be sufficiently clear, but what does one have to do to make the qi arrive? What do you do when the qi does not arrive? How can one induce the arrival of qi?

In Chapter 27 of *Directions to the Essential Methods of Acupuncture* (Iwata, 1684) there is a heading entitled "Perceiving the Coming and Going of Qi":

> This is the essence of acupuncture [that is, perceiving the coming and going of qi]. Qi refers to normal qi. Pay close attention and focus on the tip of the needle. It is vague and difficult to feel, but the coming of qi is like a fish swallowing a fishhook and it causes movements like floating and sinking. Thus, the tip of the needle moves and resistance can be felt. Do not retain the needle after the qi arrives. This is because normal qi will be dissipated. When qi does not arrive, it feels useless, like needling a piece of tofu. In this case, the qi can be made to arrive by moving the tip of the needle slightly or twisting or flicking the needle. This is known as inducing qi.

This passage suggests that qi can be made to arrive by twisting, flicking, or moving the needle a little. I have a personal example that illustrates how I get the qi to arrive. I often get a heavy sensation in the pit of my stomach (perhaps from drinking too much). My pulse is often deficient in the Liver and Kidney positions, which indicates a Liver deficiency pattern. I usually follow the principle described in Chapter 68 of the *Classic of Difficulties*, that is, needle the well point for distention in the epigastrium, and so I needle LR-1. In this one instance, however, I decide to apply the principle in chapter 69, that is, needle the mother point to tonify deficiency, and so I needle LR-8 instead. Lying on my back, I cross my left leg over my right with both knees bent at a right angle, locate LR-8 on the medial side of the left knee, and place a 30mm, No. 0 needle on this point along with the tube. Removing the tube without tapping the head of the needle, I rotate the needle back and forth with the tip resting on the skin. Immediately, my stomach begins to make sounds, and the tension in my abdomen disperses downward. All the while, I feel the arrival of qi in the fingers of my inserting hand. This seems to go on forever, as long as I keep rotating the needle.

According to some of the classics, the needle can be removed once the qi arrives. However, I continue to rotate the needle because it feels so good. I finally become tired of it and remove the needle and close the point. I go on to needle LR-8 on the right side in the same manner. When the symptom is completely resolved, however, there is no need to needle the other side. It can be considered a waste of time.

People often ask me about which side to treat when needling for the root treatment. Whether one should treat one side or both, and if one side, which side is used, the healthy side or the affected side? Some say different sides should be needled on men and women. This question can best be answered by using the analogy of blowing air into a U-shaped tube that is open on both ends. Blowing on either side moves air through the whole tube. One end serves just as well as the other.

Anyway, I needle LR-8 on the other side as well, and finally get tired of rotating the needle, so I remove it. After this, I needle CV-12 and CV-14, but in terms of effect, it really does not matter whether I do these or not. In this situation, the one needle at LR-8 on the left had effected 80 percent of the treatment, and the needle at LR-8 on the right had effected 20 percent of the treatment. The effect of a root treatment is remarkable when the treatment points are selected based on the correct pattern, and are located accurately. Being human, however, I do not always get it right. Therefore, in order to get better results, I often have to figure out symptomatic treatment strategies in addition to the root treatment.

Needling the Five-Phasic Points

When tonifying the five-phasic points of the yin meridians, the arrival of qi is felt at a much shallower depth than at other points. Needling these points is not so difficult, however, as long as one is familiar with the feeling associated with the arrival of qi. Do not tap in the needle. Just place the tube and needle on the point, remove the tube, and rotate the needle on the skin. It is best to just rotate the needle on the surface, as if doing contact needling. This, again, is what I call the super-superficial technique. It does not work very well if one tries to work in the needle as the rotations are applied. It either causes pain or you miss the sensation of the arrival of qi. As the needle is rotated on the surface, the tip of the needle will gradually begin to feel heavier. This sensation is not clear unless you remain alert and breathe slowly and quietly. So it does take some effort. Sometimes, as I rotate the needle, it starts to penetrate the skin slightly. In this case, I might add a very slight up-and-down motion to the needle, along with the rotation motion, to facilitate the arrival of qi.

Again, I quote from Yanagiya:

> When practicing this, one must be very strict about one's attention, breathing, and posture. [The area around] CV-6 in the lower abdomen must be filled and the eyes must be half closed, as if [sitting] in a Zen meditation hall. One must forget about time and fix all of one's attention on the needle. Even a mosquito, when it is about to bite, assumes a special stance, tenses its legs, places its proboscis on the skin, and inserts it gradually. It says in the ninth chapter of *Vital Axis* that 'When inserting the needle, do not look, do not listen, do not speak, and do not move. Simply pay close attention to focus on the tip of the needle to feel for the coming and going of qi.' In this way, it is pointless to talk about this [technique] without a reverent attitude of approaching the mystery of Nature. (Yanagiya, 1980)

Needling Regular Points

The arrival of qi is important for effectively needling regular points, but it is felt at a deeper level than for the five-phasic points. Take, for example, the case of myofascial back pain with pain around BL-52, and let us say that a reactive point around BL-52 needs to be needled. Before inserting the needle, I check to see which movement produces what kind of back pain. Then I palpate the most indurated point with my most sensitive fingertip. The arrival of qi will be incomplete unless the point location is precise. I use a 40mm, No. 0, stainless steel needle and tap the needle in only part way, and then remove the tube and advance the needle slowly. The trick is not to insert the needle too quickly.

Sometimes, it is difficult to determine whether the reaction is shallow or deep. Palpating the induration from the skin surface does not always give one a clear idea. Ideally, the arrival of qi should be as close to the surface as possible. Therefore, if I do not feel the arrival of qi after inserting the needle about half a unit, I withdraw the needle part way. I then apply a miniscule lifting and thrusting movement, and if I begin to feel some resistance at the tip of the needle, I start to rotate it. My rotations are only about a quarter of a turn back and forth. The speed of this rotation, however, is very fast. I go as fast as 300 turns a minute. There is no need to go quite so fast, but it seems to me that the faster the rotations, the faster the arrival of qi.

The text *Sugiyama Style of Treatment in Three Parts* briefly describes the benefit of inducing the arrival of qi:

> The benefit is, you can reduce the time it takes to give a treatment. Those who can get the arrival of qi quickly also get an effect quickly, and the condition improves more. (Sugiyama, 1682)

When I cannot get the qi to arrive close to the surface, I insert the needle a little deeper and then rotate it. If you are skilled, you can probe deeper as you rotate and lift and thrust the needle at the same time. This back and forth movement is just like boring a hole in the earth to dig a well. Pay close attention to feel for some resistance at the needle tip. Stop the lifting and thrusting motion as soon as you feel some resistance, and just rotate the needle there. This will cause the resistance to increase even more.

At this point, the patient often reports a needle sensation in the most painful or problematic place. If the patient says that the problem is somewhere else or that you are not on the right spot, you have to palpate and needle another point. Your original insertion is not in vain, however, if the point you needled was clearly an induration.

What do you do once you feel resistance around the needle? In *Directions to the Essential Methods of Acupuncture* (Iwata, 1684) it is said that the needle should be removed as soon as the qi arrives because normal qi is lost when the needle is retained. My own experience with reactive points, however, is that it is more effective to retain the needle for a short while. It is alright to retain the needle in the usual way by letting go of the needle. However, for important points, I like to retain the needle by continuing to hold the body of the needle with the supporting hand. This prevents the possibility of the patient moving and the needle tip getting off the point.

It is best not to let go of a deeply inserted, retained needle. Instead, hold the body of the needle firmly between the thumb and index finger of the supporting hand. Just holding on to the needle in this way, however, can become tedious. While waiting, you can flick the head of the needle with the pad of a finger or a fingernail. I prefer to continue rotating the needle while also adding a very small up-and-down motion. I am careful to stay on the point as I continue this subtle manipulation. I usually do this for 15 to 20 seconds, and 30 seconds when I am more thorough.

After retaining the needle this way for a minute or so, I begin to rotate the needle once more. This time, the resistance felt at the tip of the needle is gone. Even if I try to locate the resistance again, it is difficult to find. If I do not feel the arrival of qi after the above manipulation, I remove the needle and carefully palpate another point and try again.

In my experience, the frequency with which one feels the arrival of qi is greater when the needles are inserted as though only contact needling was going to be performed, that is, without intending to insert the needle. Of course, I do not seek the arrival of qi at every point I needle. As previously noted, it is better to emphasize a few points in the treatment, and so I insert the needle with great care in just a few key points. Some of my favorite symptomatic points where I seek the arrival of qi are:

• the iliac point for lower back pain
• GB-20 for dizziness
• GB-21, BL-43, and ST-12 (scalene point) for stiffness in the neck and shoulders.

In summary, the arrival of qi at regular points is usually felt as increased resistance at the tip of the needle. Also, both the patient and the practitioner often experience a pleasant sensation. In order to facilitate the arrival of qi, insert the needle gradually, stop advancing the needle as soon as some resistance is felt, and rotate the needle. This will increase the feeling of resistance at the tip of the needle. To obtain the arrival of qi even sooner, a minute lifting-and-thrusting motion can be added to the needle, along with the rotation motion. If the qi still does not arrive, remove the needle and try again, but this time, do not tap the needle in. Once you learn to feel for the arrival of qi, you can detect it even when the insertion is very superficial or the needle is not inserted at all. Take your time and pay close attention as you insert the needle in key points until you learn to feel the arrival of qi, and practice repeatedly. With enough practice, anyone can learn to feel the arrival of qi.

Conclusion

Even when the same point is needled, the degree and quality of sensation varies with the skill level of the practitioner. Thus, even if the point is located correctly, the treatment results depend on the needling technique. This can be compared to art or calligraphy where the work of an amateur and master is worlds apart even though the same materials and tools are used. This is why acupuncture is an art. This being the case, we can only needle each point with care on a daily basis to hone our skill.

There is the word *shin-gi* (heart technique) in Japan. Heart refers to a person's attitude, worldview, philosophy, or religion. It seems that very few people ask themselves fundamental questions like "Why am I living?" or "Why am I an acupuncturist?" Technique is important, but the intention behind it is even more important.

When it comes to technique, there are basically two approaches. One is the modern Western approach that includes the medical tests and physical exam techniques we use in our practice. The other is the classical Oriental approach that is recorded in many classics such as *Basic Questions* and *Classic of Difficulties*. The "technique" in these texts includes ideology, diagnosis, and treatment methods. Few acupuncturists in Japan learn the classical approach. It would be ideal if a practitioner could absorb as much of both approaches as possible. I am convinced that something new and better will emerge only from the diligent application of both approaches.

ENDNOTE

1. The following are the metric equivalents of the Japanese needle widths:

No. 02 (also called No. 00) = 0.12mm
No. 01 (also called No. 0) = 0.14mm
No. 1 = 0.16mm
No. 2 = 0.18mm
No. 3 = 0.20mm
No. 4 = 0.22mm
No. 5 = 0.24mm

APPENDIX 1

Bibliography

Primary References

Huang-Fu Mi, *Systematic Classic of Acupuncture and Moxibustion (Zhen jiu jia yi jing),* c. 259.

Hua Shou, *Elaboration of the Fourteen Meridians (Shi si jing fa hui),* 1341.

Hara Nanyō, *Clarification of Acupuncture Points (Keiketsu ikai),* 1807.

Honma Shōhaku, *Illustrated Manual to Practical Acupuncture and Moxibustion Points (Zukai shinkyū jitsuyō keiketsu gaku).* Yokosuka: Idō-No-Nippon-Sha, 1955.

Kinoshita Haruto and Shiroda Fumio, *Acupuncture Point Edition of Illustrated Guide to Oriental Medicine (Zusetsu tōyō igaku keiketsu hen).* Gakushū Kenkyū Sha, 1985.

Fukumoto Kentarō, *Location of Essential Points (Yōketsu no shuketsu).* Japan Meridian Therapy Association, 1986.

Chinese References

Anonymous, *Basic Questions (Su wen),* c. 1st century B.C.

Anonymous, *Vital Axis, (Ling shu),* c. 1st century B.C.

Bian Que (attribution), *Classic of Difficulties (Nan jing),* c. 2nd century A.D.

Gao Wu, *Gatherings from Outstanding Acupuncturists (Zhen jiu ju ying),* 1529.

Ge Hong, *Handbook of Emergency Prescriptions (Zhou hou bei ji fang),* 340.

Gai Guo-Cai, *Acupuncture Point Diagnosis (Tsubo shindanhō,* a Chinese text translated into Japanese by Mitsutane Sugi). Yokosuka: Idō-No-Nippon-Sha, 1984.

Hao Jin-Kai, *Atlas of Off-Meridian Miscellaneous Points for Acupuncture (Zhen jiu jing wai qi xue tu pu).* Nantong: Nantong Stationary & Publishing Co., 1973.

Huang-Fu Mi, *Systematic Classic on Acupuncture and Moxibustion (Zhen jiu jia yi jing),* c. 259.

Hua Shou, *Elaboration of the Fourteen Meridians (Shi si jing fa hui),* 1341.

Li Ding, *Acupuncture and Moxibustion Point Dictionary (Zhen jiu jing xue ci dian).* Tianjin: Tianjin Institute of Traditional Chinese Medicine, 1986.

Shanghai Institute of Chinese Medicine, *Acupuncture: A Comprehensive Text (Zhen jiu xue).* Shanghai: Renmin Weisheng Chubanshe, 1974; 2nd Japanese ed., Tokyo: Kenkodo Publishing, 1977.

Sun Si-Miao, *Prescriptions Worth a Thousand Gold Pieces (Qian jin yao fang),* c. 700.

Wang Shu-He, *Pulse Classic (Mai jing),* 280.

Wang Wei-Yi, *Illustrated Manual of the Acupuncture and Moxibustion Points on the Bronze Figure (Tong ren shu xue zen jiu tu jing),* 1027.

Wang Zhi-Zhong, *Compilation of Resources of Acupuncture and Moxibustion (Zhen jiu zi sheng jing),* 1165.

Xu Feng, *Complete Compilation of Acupuncture and Moxibustion Classics (Zhen jiu da quan)*, 1439.

Yang Ji-Zhou, *Compendium of Acupuncture and Moxibustion (Zhen jiu da cheng)*, 1601.

Zhang Jie-Bin, *Classification of the Classics (Lei jing)*, 1624.

Zheng Kui-Shan, *Collection of the Finest in Acupuncture and Moxibustion (Zhen jiu ji jin)*. Shizen-sha, 1983.

Zhang Zhong-Jing, *Essentials from the Golden Cabinet (Jin kui yao lue)*, early 3rd century A.D.

Japanese References

Akabane Kōhei, *Acupuncture and Moxibustion Treatment Based on Measurement of Heat Sensitivity (Chinetsu kando sokutei niyoru shinkyū chiryōhō)*. Yokosuka: Idō-No-Nippon-Sha, 1954.

Akabane Kōhei, *Intradermal Needle Technique (Hinaishin-hō)*. Yokosuka: Idō-No-Nippon-Sha, 1964.

Araki Masatane, *Kampō Therapy (Kampō chiryō)*. Tokyo: Iwasaki Shoten, 1957.

Birch, Stephen and Ida Junko, *Japanese Acupuncture: A Clinical Guide*. Brookline, MA: Paradigm Publications, 1998.

Chikuta Takichi, *Secrets of Practical Nursing Care in the Home (Katei-ni-okeru jissai kango-no-hiketsu)*, rev. ed. Sanjuen-sha, 1954.

Fukaya Isaburō, *Stories from a Moxibustion Practice (Rinshō kyūdō yoroku)*. Shinkyū-no Sekai, 1966.

Fukumoto Kentarō, *Location of Essential Points (Yōketsu no shuketsu)*. Japan Meridian Therapy Association, 1986.

Hara Nanyō, *Clarification of Acupuncture Points (Keiketsu ikai)*, 1807.

Hongō Masatoyo, *A Precious Record of Acupuncture and Moxibustion (Shinky chōhōki)*, 1718. Reprinted by Japan Meridian Therapy Association, 1982.

Honma Shōhaku, *Discourse on Meridian Therapy (Keiraku chiryō kōwa)*. Yokosuka: Idō-No-Nippon-Sha, 1949.

Honma Shōhaku, *Illustrated Guide to Practical Acupuncture and Moxibustion Points (Zukai shinkyū jitsuyō keiketsu gaku)*. Yokosuka: Idō-No-Nippon Company, 1955.

Honma Shōhaku, *Study of the Classic of Difficulties (Nangyo no kenkyu)*. Yokosuka: Idō-No-Nippon-Sha, 1965.

Irie Seiji, *Illustrated Guide to Fukayaōì Moxibustion Techniques (Zusetsu fukaya kyūhō)*. Shizen-sha, 1980.

Inoue Keiri, *Nanjing Lectures* (audiotapes). Toyohari Medical Association, 1965.

Ishizaka Sōkei, *Special Stories of Acupuncture and Moxibustion (Shinkyū meiwa)*, 1860. Reprinted by Idō-No-Nippon-Sha, 1957.

Ishizaka Sōtetsu, *Concise Discourse on Acupuncture and Moxibustion (Shikyu setsuyaku)*, 1812. Reprinted by Seibun-dō.

Ishizuka Bunjō, *Difficult to Learn Point Locations (Kongaku keppō)*, 1835.

Iwata Risai, *Directions to the Essential Methods of Acupuncture (Shinkyu youhou shinan)*, 1684.

Kinoshita Haruto, *Treatment of Sciatica (Zakotsushinkei-no-chiryō)*. Tōyō Igaku Sha, 1968.

Kinoshita Haruto and Shiroda Fumio, *Acupuncture Point Edition of Illustrated Guide to Oriental Medicine (Zusetsu tōyō igaku keiketsu hen)*. Gakushū Kenkyū Sha, 1985.

Kosoto Yō, *The Pulse Classic: An Outline (Myakuron: sōsetsu)*, vol. 8 of *Oriental Medicine Compendium*. Toyo Igaku Kenkyū-kai, 1981.

Manaka Yoshio with Itaya Kazuko & Birch, Stephen, *Chasing the Dragon's Tail*. Brookline, MA: Paradigm Publications, 1995.

Manase Dōsan, *Newly Compiled Addition to the Secrets of Pulse Diagnosis (Shinsen zōho myakuron kuketsu)*, 1578. Reprinted by Japan Meridian Therapy Association, 1982.

Maruyama Masao, *The Study of Acupuncture and Moxibustion and the Classics (Shinkyū igaku to koten no kenkyū)*. Tokyo: Sōgen-sha, 1977.

Mori Hidetarō, *Study of Acupuncture Point Anatomy (Kaibō keiketsugaku)*. Yokosuka: Idō-No-Nippon-Sha, 1981.

Mubunsai, *Compilation of the Secrets of Acupuncture (Shindō hiketsushū)*, 1685. Reprinted by Seibundo Oriental Medical Publications, 1980.

Nakamura Yaeko, Shudo Denmei, "One-Needle Technique for Rejuvenation" *(Waka-gaeri-no-ippon-shin)*. *Journal of Japanese Acupuncture and Moxibustion* 35; 381, May, 1976.

Nanzandō Medical Dictionary. Tokyo: Nanzandō Company, 1978.

Okabe Sodō, *Acupuncture by Meridian Therapy (Shinkyū keiraku chiryō)*. Tokyo: Sekibundō, 1974.

Okabe Sodō, *The Essence of Acupuncture Therapy (Shinkyū chiryō no shinzui)*. Tokyo: Sekibundō, 1983.

Okabe Sodō, "Introduction to Meridian Therapy: Diagnosis" *(Keiraku chiryō nyu-mon: shindanhen)*. *Oriental Medical Journal* 11(2), Feb., 1944.

Okamoto Ippō, *Guide to the Secrets of Moxibustion (Kyūhō kuketsu shinan)*, 1685.

Okamoto Ippō, *Japanese Commentaries on Elaboration of the Fourteen Meridians (Jyushi keiraku hakki wakai)*, 1693.

Shibasaki Michizō, *Compendium of Acupuncture and Moxibustion Medicine (Shinkyū igaku taikei)*. Yūkun-sha, 1979.

Shiroda Bunshi, *Basic Study of Acupuncture and Moxibustion Therapy (Shinkyū chiryō kisogaku)*. Yokosuka: Idō-No-Nippon-Sha, 1940.

Shiroda Fumio, *Acupuncture and Moxibustion Point Dictionary (Shinkyū keiketsu jiten)*. Tōyō Igaku Shuppan, 1985.

Shudō Denmei, "Effective Points for Treatment of Low Back Pain" *(Yōtsu-no-chiryō-ni-kiku-tsubo)*, *Journal of Japanese Acupuncture and Moxibustion* 34; 375, June, 1975.

Shudō Denmei, *Japanese Classical Acupuncture: Introduction to Meridian Therapy.* Seattle: Eastland Press, 1990.

Suganuma Shūkei, *Rules of Acupuncture (Shinkyū soku)*,1766.

Sugiyama Waichi, *Sugiyama Style of Treatment in Three Parts (Sugiyama sanbusho)*, 1682. Reprinted by Idō-No-Nippon-Sha, 1976.

Taki Motokata, "Unusual Manifestations of Disease" *(Shinbyō kigai)*, in *Nippon Kanpō Fukushin Sōsho (Japan Herbology Abdominal Diagnosis Digest)*, 1843.

Yamashita Makoto, *Illustrated Clinical Meridians and Acupuncture Points (Rinshō keiraku keiketsu zukai)*. Ishiyaku Publishing Company, 1972.

Yanagiya Sorei, *Revised Guide to Shu Points of the Fourteen Meridians (Kōtei jyūshikei yuketsu gaku)*. Handaya, 1948.

Yanagiya Sorei, *Guide to Secret One-Needle Technique (Hihō ipponshin densho)*. Yokosuka: Idō-No-Nippon-Sha, 1955.

Yanagiya Sorei, *Simple Diagnosis Without Questioning (Kanmei fumon shinsatsuhō)*. Ishiyama Shinkyū Igaku Sha, 1976.

Yanagiya Sorei, *Illustrated Guide to Acupuncture and Moxibustion Techniques (Zusetsu shinyu jitsugi)*. Idō-No-Nippon-Sha, 7th ed., 1977.

Yanagiya Sorei, compiled by Yanagiya Sei-itsu, *The Gate to Acupuncture and Moxibustion Techniques (Shinkyu ijyutsu no mon)*. Ishiyama Shinkyu Igaku Sha, 1980.

Yokota Kampū, *Lectures on Pathways of Meridians (Keiraku ryuchū kōgi)*. Yokosuka: Idō-No-Nippon-Sha, 1995.

APPENDIX 2

Point Index by Meridian

T HE WORLD HEALTH ORGANIZATION (WHO) designation or miscellaneous name for each acupuncture point is followed by one to three stars indicating the frequency of use of that point by the author (see Chapter 2), the Japanese/Chinese transliteration, and page number in this book.

Lung

LU-1 (★★) *chū-fu/zhōng fǔ, 110*
LU-5 (★★★) *shaku-taku/chǐ zé, 149*
LU-6 (★★) *kō-sai/kǒng zuì, 147*
LU-7 (★) *rek-ketsu/lìe quē, 146*
LU-8 (★★) *kei-kyo/jīng qú, 145*
LU-9 (★★★) *tai-en/tài yuān, 144*
LU-10 (★) *gyo-sai/yú jì, 143*
LU-11 (★★) *shō-shō/shào shāng, 141*

Large Intestine

LI-2 (★) *ji-kan/èr jiān, 160*
LI-4 (★★) *gō-koku/hé gǔ, 163*
LI-6 (★) *hen-reki/piān lì, 164*

Heart

HT-3 (★) *shō-kai/shào hǎi, 160*
HT-6 (★) *in-geki/yīn xī, 158*
HT-7 (★) *shin-mon/shén mén, 158*
HT-9 (★) *shō-shō/shào chōng, 155*

Small Intestine

SI-1 (★★) *shō-taku/shào zé, 170*
SI-3 (★★★) *kō-kei/hòu xī, 172*
SI-9 (★★) *ken-tei/jiān zhēn, 61*
SI-11 (★★★) *ten-sō/tiān zōng, 60*

Bladder

BL-1 (★) *sei-mei/jīng míng, 39*
BL-2 (★★★) *san-chiku/zǎn zhú, 37*
BL-3 (★) *bi-shō/méi chōng, 23*
BL-10 (★★) *ten-chū/tiān zhù, 24*
BL-12 (★★) *fū-mon/fēng mén, 73*
BL-13 (★★★) *hai-yu/fèi shū, 74*
BL-14 (★★★) *ketsu-in-yu/jué yīn shū, 77*
BL-15 (★★★) *shin-yu/xīn shū, 77*
BL-17 (★★) *kaku-yu/gé shū, 80*
BL-18 (★★★) *kan-yu/gān shū, 81*
BL-19 (★★) *tan-yu/dǎn shū, 82*
BL-20 (★★★) *hi-yu/pí shū, 83*
BL-21 (★★) *i-yu/wèi shū, 84*
BL-22 (★★) *san-shō-yu/sān jiāo shū, 85*
BL-23 (★★★) *jin-yu/shèn shū, 86*
BL-25 (★★) *dai-chō-yu/dà cháng shū, 87*
BL-27 (★) *shō-chō-yu/xiǎo cháng shū, 91*
BL-32 (★) *ji-ryō/cì liáo, 92*
BL-35 (★) *e-yō/huì yáng, 94*
BL-37 (★★) *in-mon/yīn mén, 225*
BL-39 (★) *i-yō/wěi yáng, 225*
BL-40 (★★) *i-chū/wěi zhōng, 222*
BL-42 (★) *haku-ko/pò hù, 96*

TB-17 （★★） *ei-fū/yì fēng, 33*
TB-20 （★） *kaku-son/jiǎo sūn, 32*
TB-23 （★） *shi-chiku-kū/sī zhú kōng, 47*

Gallbladder

GB-1 （★） *dō-ji-ryō/tóng zǐ liáo, 47*
GB-2 （★★） *chō-e/tīng huì, 49*
GB-3 （★） *jō-kan/shàng guān, 50*
GB-5 （★★） *ken-ro/xuán lú, 51*
GB-6 （★★） *ken-ri/xuán lí, 52*
GB-11 （★） *atama-kyō-in/tóu qiào yīn, 34*
GB-12 （★★） *kan-kotsu/wán gǔ, 34*
GB-14 （★） *yō-haku/yáng bái, 44*
GB-20 （★★★） *fū-chi/fēng chí, 27*
GB-21 （★★★） *ken-sei/jiān jǐng, 57*
GB-24 （★） *jitsu-getsu/rì yuè, 135*
GB-25 （★） *kei-mon/jīng mén, 139*
GB-29 （★） *kyo-ryō/jū liáo, 190*
GB-30 （★★★） *kan-chō/huán tiào, 213*
GB-34 （★★） *yō-ryō-sen/yáng líng quán, 211*
GB-38 （★★★） *yō-ho/yáng fǔ, 210*
GB-39 （★★） *ken-shō/xuán zhōng, 210*
GB-40 （★） *kyū-kyo/qīu xū, 208*

Liver

LR-1 （★★★） *dai-ton/dà dūn, 183*
LR-2 （★★） *kō-kan/xíng jiān, 185*
LR-3 （★★） *tai-shō/tài chōng, 185*
LR-4 （★★） *chū-hō/zhōng fēng, 186*
LR-5 （★） *rei-kō/lǐ gōu, 187*
LR-8 （★★★） *kyoku-sen/qǔ quán, 188*
LR-13 （★★） *shō-mon/zhāng mén, 135*
LR-14 （★★） *ki-mon/qī mén, 132*

Governor Vessel

GV-2 （★） *yō-yu/yāo shū, 72*

General Index

——— **M**